The I.B.S. Diet

The I.B.S. Diet

Sarah Brewer MD *and*

Michelle Berriedale-Johnson

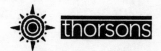

Thorsons
An Imprint of HarperCollins*Publishers*
77–85 Fulham Palace Road
Hammersmith, London W6 8JB

The website address is: www.thorsonselement.com

and *Thorsons* are trademarks of
HarperCollins*Publishers* Limited

First published as *Eat to Beat I.B.S.* by Thorsons 2002
This edition 2004

10 9 8 7 6 5 4 3 2 1

A catalogue record for this book
is available from the British Library

ISBN 0 00 715811 4

Printed in Great Britain by
Clays Ltd, St Ives plc

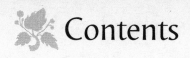# Contents

How to use this book

The first part of *The I.B.S. Diet* tells you all about the condition, its symptoms and how you might be investigated and treated by your doctor. The second part tells you how you can help yourself through relatively simple diet and lifestyle changes. Chapter 5 entitled Eat to Beat I.B.S. gives an overview of dietary changes that might help, while Chapters 6 to 10 look at common triggers such as dietary fibre, wheat, dairy products and covers food intolerance and Candida.

Once you have decided which types of food to avoid, or include in your diet, the delicious recipes compiled by Michelle Berriedale-Johnson will help you achieve this as simply as possible. A number of food and herbal supplements can help relieve symptoms and these are covered in Chapter 17, while lifestyle changes can be found in Chapter 18, with useful contact addresses detailed in the appendix.

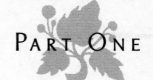

PART ONE

The Facts about I.B.S.

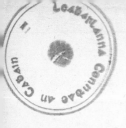

CHAPTER 1

What is I.B.S.?

Irritable Bowel Syndrome is the most common condition to affect the gut. At least a third of the population is affected at some time during their life, even if only mildly, and one in seven is affected badly enough to consult a doctor. As many other bowel conditions can cause similar symptoms initially, I.B.S. is not a diagnosis you should make yourself. Once your doctor has confirmed you have I.B.S., however, you can improve your symptoms and transform your quality of life by eating a bowel-friendly diet, based on recipes such as those found in this book. You can also make effective changes to your lifestyle (*see Chapter 18*), and obtain benefit from a number of food supplements (*see Chapter 17*).

I.B.S. is a problem of bowel function rather than structure. As a result, there is nothing abnormal to find during investigations. The diagnosis is therefore made on the basis of symptoms alone, using a system known as the Rome II Criteria, which were updated in 1999.

For your doctor to diagnose Irritable Bowel Syndrome, you must have had at least 12 weeks (which need not be consecutive) in the preceding 12 months of abdominal discomfort or pain that has two of three features:

* Relieved by opening your bowels; and/or
* Onset associated with a change in frequency of stool; and/or
* Onset associated with a change in form (appearance) of stool

The following symptoms also add up to support the diagnosis of I.B.S.:

1 Fewer than three bowel movements a week
2 More than three bowel movements a day
3 Hard or lumpy stools
4 Loose (mushy) or watery stools
5 Straining during a bowel movement
6 Urgency (having to rush to have a bowel movement)
7 Feeling of incomplete bowel movement
8 Passing mucus (white material) during a bowel movement
9 Abdominal fullness, bloating or swelling

Typically, motions are small, frequent, pencil-like, or resemble rabbit droppings, but those with the diarrhoea-predominant form of I.B.S. have one or more of symptoms 2, 4 or 6 and none of symptoms 1, 3 or 5, while those with the constipation-predominant type have one or more of symptoms 1, 3 or 5 and none of 2, 4 or 6.

Who gets it?

I.B.S. is traditionally said to affect young and middle-aged adults. Symptoms usually start between the ages of 15 and 40, with the commonest presentation being between the ages of 30 and 40. It can, however, affect anyone at any age, and recent studies have suggested that more people are affected in the 45–65 age range than in younger age groups. Symptoms can also occur in children.

I.B.S. is often described as a problem affecting women rather than men. Some studies suggest that twice as many women as men are affected, although others have found that men are just as likely to have symptoms of I.B.S. as women, but are less likely to consult their doctor. As a result, two out of every three people referred to hospital clinics and diagnosed as having I.B.S. are female. This led many researchers to the opinion that I.B.S. was a psychosomatic problem linked with hysteria and neurosis. More enlightened scientists, however, started wondering about the role of the female hormones oestrogen and progesterone (*see page 15*).

How do symptoms occur?

I.B.S. seems to be linked with abnormal or exaggerated bowel movements and muscular spasm.

The intestines are made up of a long tube which contracts in ordered waves to push food through whilst nutrients and water are absorbed. In a healthy bowel, the contents are propelled downwards smoothly. In I.B.S. sufferers, however, the passage is irregular, leading to recurrent symptoms of bloating, wind, constipation, diarrhoea and/or pain.

Imagine the gut as a long, flexible, plastic tube filled with porridge and closed off at one end. If you picked up the closed end of the tube and squeezed it with both hands, the porridge contents would be forced further down the tube. If you then let go with the hand nearest the closed end, and squeezed on the other side of the hand still gripping the tube, you would force the porridge down even further. If you repeated this movement, systematically releasing one hand at a time and squeezing further and further down the tube, you would eventually end up with a pile of porridge on the floor and a relatively clean, empty tube. This represents normal bowel movement.

Now imagine a similar tube filled with porridge, again held with both hands near the closed end. Instead of smoothly constricting the tube in an ordered wave down its length, let go of the tube with one hand and squeeze it anywhere you like along its length. Repeat this random squeeze on the tube with alternate hands. You will eventually end up with some porridge on the floor, but the tube is likely to stay relatively full, with porridge built up in some areas, and squeezed out in others to resemble a string of sausages. This is similar to what may happen with I.B.S.

In a normally-functioning bowel, smooth muscular waves of constriction run down the gut in an ordered fashion. A wave of constriction is preceded by a wave of relaxation and this pushes the bowel contents downwards. This characteristic movement of the bowel is known as peristalsis.

In I.B.S., it is thought that peristalsis becomes disordered. Waves of constriction and relaxation become separated and random parts of the bowel may go into cramp. If waves of constriction are speeded up, diarrhoea occurs. If waves of constriction are slowed down, or become irregular, constipation occurs, and this is made worse if the bowel goes into cramp. If the bowel stays constricted, and only dilates occasionally, the contents may become concentrated into thin ribbons, or separated into pellets like rabbit droppings. If constriction is persistent, and bowel movements infrequent, the contents harden up as more water than normal is reabsorbed. This can lead to hardened, concrete-like motions, with or without mucus.

If the bowel dilates between cramp attacks, two things can happen. If the gut is full, the contents become unusually large and difficult to push out; but if the gut is empty, it can fill with wind to cause bloating, stretch pains plus embarrassing rumblings and flatulence.

Your digestive system

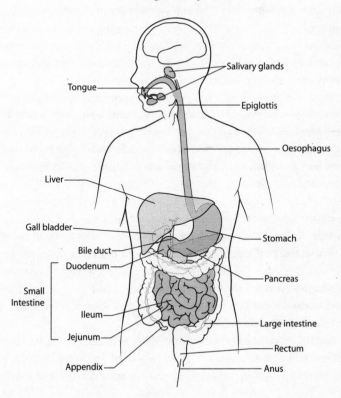

What are the symptoms of I.B.S.?

The symptoms of I.B.S. vary from person to person and may come and go over a period of time. The bowel symptoms that occur most often include:

- Lower abdominal pain or discomfort
- Bloating
- Wind, with distension of abdomen, rumbling (borborygmi) and flatulence
- Constipation
- Diarrhoea
- Having to rush to the loo (urgency)
- Altered stool frequency
- Altered stool form
- Altered stool passage with feelings of incomplete emptying
- Mucus
- Nausea
- Upper abdominal pain
- Rectal pain

Researchers at the Central Middlesex Hospital NHS Trust in the UK have identified three different types of I.B.S. based on the main symptoms experienced by sufferers. These are Spastic Colon Syndrome, Functional Diarrhoea Syndrome and Primary Foregut Motility Disorder.

SPASTIC COLON SYNDROME

Spastic Colon Syndrome is identified where the onset of lower abdominal pain is associated with:

- Passing looser stools than normal
- Abdominal distension
- Relief of symptoms on opening the bowel
- Feelings of incomplete evacuation of the bowel
- Mucus in the stools

Loose motions and constipation tend to alternate. Women suffering from this form of I.B.S. are more likely to report difficulty in passing urine and gynaecological problems, with I.B.S. symptoms being worse at certain times of the menstrual cycle. Spastic Colon Syndrome is the classic form of I.B.S., due to abnormal contractions of the large bowel. Constipation is usually a major feature of spastic colon syndrome, and tends to respond to an increased fibre diet. Smooth muscle relaxant drugs and antispasmodics are usually helpful too.

FUNCTIONAL DIARRHOEA SYNDROME
Functional Diarrhoea Syndrome is associated with:

- Increased frequency of bowel movements
- Urgency (having to rush to the bathroom)
- Passing several stools in rapid succession, often in the morning
- Stools that characteristically become looser throughout the day

Sufferers are frequently left exhausted, and the rapidity with which the bowels have to be opened can mean they are housebound or unable to travel far. This form of I.B.S. is likely to be made worse by following a high-fibre diet, but will usually respond to treatment with anti-diarrhoeal drugs such as loperamide or Imodium.

PRIMARY FOREGUT MOTILITY DISORDER
Primary Foregut Motility Disorder is linked with:

- Abdominal pain, usually on the right side
- Bloating, which may be so severe that you have to wear loose clothing or even different-sized clothes on various days
- Feeling full after eating only a small amount of food
- Poor appetite
- Weight loss (sometimes)

There is usually no significant disturbance of bowel habit in this form of I.B.S., so diarrhoea and constipation are not a major problem. This disorder is believed to result from abnormal contraction of the small intestine rather than the colon. It seems to affect women more than men. Unfortunately, the condition can be difficult to treat, although drugs that stimulate and regulate intestinal movement may help.

This is not a foolproof classification of I.B.S. types. Many sufferers cannot fit their symptoms neatly into one group. Chapter 3 looks in more detail at the symptoms of I.B.S.

CHAPTER 2

Causes of I.B.S.

Different people find that different factors can trigger their symptoms of I.B.S. A particular incident may bring symptoms on for the first time, or recurrent symptoms may be linked with some aspect of your diet or lifestyle. Common trigger factors that may bring on symptoms in people with a predisposition to I.B.S. include:

* Gastroenteritis
* Taking antibiotics
* Taking certain drugs
* Smoking cigarettes
* The menstrual cycle
* Lack of sleep
* Stress
* Candida yeast infection
* Eating certain foods

Gastroenteritis

Food poisoning, or gastroenteritis, is caused by eating or drinking contaminated food or liquids. Foods that have been improperly cooked or reheated are particularly risky as they may contain pathogenic (disease-causing) bacteria, viruses or pre-formed toxins. Symptoms usually appear within 30 minutes in the cases of chemical poisoning, between 1 and 12 hours if the illness is due to bacterial toxins, and between 12 and 48 hours if it results from a bacterial or viral infection. Most cases of food poisoning cause stomach pains, vomiting and/or diarrhoea, which usually improve within a few days.

More serious cases may cause fever and loss of blood in the motions – a condition referred to as dysentery.

Diarrhoea affects up to half of those visiting tropical regions. Surprisingly, even 10 per cent of visitors to European resorts also succumb. The commonest bacteria involved are toxin-producing strains of E. coli, campylobacter, salmonella and shigella, which can cause severe gastroenteritis with abdominal pain, vomiting and diarrhoea. Most healthy people will have an unpleasant time as a result, but will recover with proper treatment.

Symptoms of I.B.S. often seem to come on or become worse after a bout of gastroenteritis. This was first noticed in the 1960s, but researchers are still unclear why it happens. The most likely explanation is that the presence of altered bacteria in the bowel leads to an imbalance that affects bowel movement in some way. It may cause inflammation, which irritates nerve endings, or increase the leakiness of the bowel wall. By letting incompletely-digested food particles through into the circulation, gastroenteritis may trigger a food sensitivity that lasts beyond the duration of the original infection. It may also encourage sensitivity to chemicals produced by Candida yeast cells (see Chapter 9).

In 1994, a study of 38 victims of an outbreak of salmonella food poisoning found that, during the following year, almost a third went on to develop recurrent bowel symptoms consistent with I.B.S. Interestingly, five times as many women as men developed I.B.S. In most cases, both male and female sufferers developed intermittent diarrhoea and bowel urgency – features of Functional Diarrhoea Syndrome. In general, those with the worst symptoms of gastroenteritis (diarrhoea lasting more than seven days plus vomiting, leading to weight loss) were more likely to develop I.B.S. than those with milder symptoms. They were also the ones who took longer to recover their appetite, weight and energy levels.

Another study looked at 75 patients who developed gastroenteritis from various organisms that was bad enough for them to be admitted to hospital. Of these, 22 (29 per cent) had symptoms three months later that were consistent with I.B.S. Nine out of ten of these were still suffering after six months, and three-quarters still had I.B.S. problems one year later. As in the first study, those with the worst symptoms (diarrhoea lasting longer, with abdominal pain and mucus in the stools) were more likely to develop I.B.S.

There is undoubtedly a link between bowel infection and inflammation and subsequent intestinal problems with pain, diarrhoea and bloating. Symptoms that improve after a few months may be due to a temporary lactase enzyme deficiency (*see page 83*). Those lasting longer may be due to other as yet unexplained changes in bowel function that may have triggered I.B.S.

In the second of the above studies, the researchers also assessed the psychological profile of the 75 patients admitted to hospital with gastroenteritis. They found that those who were most anxious, and who reported the most unexplained non-intestinal symptoms during their admission to hospital, were also more likely to develop I.B.S. later, suggesting that psychological factors do increase the risk of developing I.B.S. after a severe bowel infection. This may be linked with the known damping down effects of stress on the immune system and the effects of stress hormones on bowel function. This in turn may slow down recovery from the illness and result in a longer, more severe bout of illness (*see 'Stress', page 208*).

Simple tips for avoiding bacterial gastroenteritis at home include:

* Wash hands thoroughly after visiting the bathroom, before preparing foods and again before eating.
* Keep your kitchen clean and dry.
* Keep pets out of the kitchen at all times.
* Keep separate chopping boards for cooked meat, raw meat and for other produce such as vegetables.
* Keep food refrigerated to help prevent bacterial growth. A rise in temperature from just 4°C to 8°C increases bacterial growth by as much as 65 per cent.
* Make sure your fridge is keeping food properly chilled with fridge temperature below 5°C and freezer temperature below −18°C.
* If using a lunch box, select one designed to keep packed food fridge-fresh for up to six hours. They contain an ice-pack that you freeze overnight, which slots into the lunch box with the dual

purpose of separating drink and yoghurt from crushable sandwiches and fruit.

* Clean your fridge regularly and throw away all foods past their use-by date.
* Store raw meat at the bottom of the fridge, covered, and separate from cooked foods.
* Defrost frozen produce thoroughly before cooking.
* Reheating food, or only partially cooking products, encourages bacterial growth. Make sure all hot food is cooked thoroughly and served piping hot rather than merely warm.
* Take a probiotic supplement *(see page 190)*.

To help avoid upset stomachs abroad:

* Only use safe water for drinking, brushing your teeth, preparing food or cooking, such as water from sealed bottles that you have opened yourself, carbonated water (which is less likely to have been filled from a tap than still water), water that has been recently boiled or water sterilized with purification tablets. Lightweight or travel-sized pump-action water filters can provide between 50 and 200 litres of safe drinking water.
* Only use ice cubes made with safe water.
* Avoid green salads, uncooked vegetables and fruits that cannot be peeled.
* Avoid unpasteurized milk – boil if you are unsure.
* Avoid ice creams from unreliable sources.
* Wash hands thoroughly before eating.
* Avoid food exposed to the sun or to flies.
* Avoid snacks bought from roadside vendors.
* Sea, river and swimming pool water may be contaminated. Keep your head out of the water and try not to swallow any. If water looks obviously murky, don't go swimming.
* Take a probiotic supplement *(see page 190)*.

You can also help boost your natural immunity to harmful bacterial infections by:

- Eating a healthy, wholefood diet.
- Eating oily fish (e.g. salmon, mackerel, herring, sardines) regularly.
- Avoiding excess stress.
- Taking regular exercise.
- Getting a regular good night's sleep.
- Taking a complete vitamin and mineral supplement.
- Taking herbal supplements containing Echinacea or Siberian ginseng (*see Chapter 17*).

Taking antibiotics

Antibiotics are drugs that kill or inactivate bacteria. They work in two main ways:

1 By punching holes in bacterial cell walls so they absorb water and burst (penicillins and cephalosporins), or
2 By interfering with bacterial protein production (e.g. tetracyclines, macrolides, aminoglycosides).

Unfortunately, antibiotics kill good bacteria as well as bad. This can lead to a bacterial imbalance in the intestines. After the original infection has been dealt with, you may still be left with a bacterial imbalance as less desirable organisms – including yeasts – flourish at the expense of others. This is known as gut dysbiosis and can affect the normal process of fermentation in the colon and change the amount and composition of bowel gases produced. Taking antibiotics often leads to diarrhoea as a direct result of these artificial changes in gut bacteria, and may trigger symptoms of I.B.S. in some people. However, in the two studies mentioned in the section on gastroenteritis above, there did not seem to be an increased risk of developing I.B.S. if the original bout of food poisoning was treated with antibiotics.

While taking a course of antibiotics, it is important to replenish the bowel with 'friendly bacteria', which will help damp down bacterial imbalances. You can do this by eating live (unpasteurized) bio yoghurt containing organisms such as *Lactobacillus acidophilus* or by taking a probiotic supplement (*see page 190*). Many I.B.S. sufferers claim that eating bio yoghurt every day helps to keep their symptoms under control, whether they have recently taken antibiotics or not.

Taking certain drugs

As well as antibiotics, many other drugs can also affect bowel function. These include:

- Laxatives
- Aspirin-like drugs (e.g. salicylic acid, ibuprofen)
- Opiate painkillers (especially opiates such as codeine phosphate and morphine)
- Antacids (especially aluminium-based ones)
- Acid-reducing drugs (e.g. H2 antagonists such as cimetidine)
- Beta-blockers (e.g. propranolol, atenolol)
- Tricyclic antidepressants (e.g. amitriptyline)
- Calcium antagonists (e.g. nifedipine)
- Iron preparations
- Steroids
- Hormonal methods of contraception
- Sleeping tablets
- Most illegal drugs
- Alcohol
- Nicotine *(see 'Smoking Cigarettes', below)*

These drugs can affect bowel movement – speeding it up or slowing it down. They can also affect gastrointestinal secretions, disrupt mucus production, affect bowel bacteria or have a direct irritant effect on the bowel wall. If you suffer from I.B.S., it is wise to avoid taking all but the most necessary medications.

Smoking cigarettes

Some of the nerve endings in the bowel can be stimulated by nicotine. Exposure to nicotine causes an initial burst of electrical activity in these nerve endings and then blocks them temporarily so that their activity becomes less than normal. This interferes with normal bowel function and the contraction of smooth muscle cells in the gut wall. Many people with I.B.S. find that exposure to cigarette smoke – even passively – can cause flushing, intestinal cramps, nausea and diarrhoea. If exposure is prolonged, it may lead to constipation. If you suffer from I.B.S., it is worth trying to stop smoking and avoid smoke-laden atmospheres.

The menstrual cycle

Although I.B.S. affects men as well as women, there are differences in bowel function between the sexes that may be linked to reproductive hormones:

* Bloating is more common in women than men
* Bowel transit time (time taken for food to pass through the gut) is slower in women, especially during the second half of the menstrual cycle
* Women excrete less bile acid than men and may digest their food less well

Researchers have now found receptors for the two main female sex hormones, oestrogen and progesterone, in the smooth muscle cells lining the small intestines and colon. These receptors seem to be found in similar numbers to those present in breast tissue, and it is likely that they are there for a purpose. It may well be that sex hormones help to regulate gut function. During the second half of the menstrual cycle, for example, when progesterone levels are naturally high, the time taken for food to pass through the gut may be almost twice as long as during the first half of the cycle.

Oestrogen is known to have an effect on smooth muscle cells in artery walls, helping to keep them elastic, while progesterone has a relaxant effect on smooth muscle cells lining the bowel and urinary system. This is why constipation and urinary tract infections are more common during pregnancy when progesterone levels are high. It seems reasonable to assume that these female hormones may also be linked with I.B.S. symptoms in women. Women with constipation, for example, often find that their symptoms are significantly better just before and during a period, when progesterone levels fall. Other symptoms, such as pain due to spasms, may become worse at this stage of the menstrual cycle. This exacerbation of symptoms does not seem to be linked with any particular psychological or emotional traits or the mood swings of premenstrual syndrome.

The effects of sex hormones on bowel emptying, bile acid secretion and I.B.S. are currently under further investigation. One theory is that the normal bacteria present in the colon are sensitive to human sex hormones and to plant hormones (e.g. phytoestrogens and isoflavones) and other substances released during the digestion of certain foods (*see list at beginning of Chapter 5, page 52*). This may change the normal fermentation processes occurring in the bowel at different times of the menstrual cycle and alter the quantity and composition of gases produced.

Yet more evidence of a role for female sex hormones comes from the fact that women are more likely to develop symptoms of I.B.S. if they have had a hysterectomy. On average, one in ten women develops problems soon after the operation. One study compared women who had undergone a hysterectomy with a similar group who had not had the operation. It found that those who had undergone surgery were more likely to:

* Consider themselves constipated
* Defecate less often
* Strain during defecation
* Experience abdominal bloating
* Have feelings of incomplete evacuation of the bowels
* Pass lumpy motions
* Have longer bowel transit times, especially in women over the age of 50

This study suggests that having a hysterectomy can affect the function of the colon and rectum – and may possibly trigger I.B.S. in some women.

Lack of sleep

Lack of sleep can make the symptoms of I.B.S. significantly worse. Research suggests that the severity of morning symptoms is closely linked to the quality of sleep the night before. Poor sleep may affect the way the brain produces chemicals such as melatonin, ACTH and adrenaline. An imbalance or overproduction of these hormones can affect gut movement. Lack of sleep also causes physical and emotional stress. This leads to raised levels of stress hormones such as adrenaline, which can affect the gut.

Stress

Stress has long been known to make the symptoms of I.B.S. worse, although there is little evidence that it can cause I.B.S. in the first place. Many sufferers state quite firmly that the only stress in their life comes from having the symptoms of I.B.S. – without these, their life would be relative bliss.

When we are experiencing stress, the body releases powerful chemicals (such as adrenaline, neuropeptide Y, somatostatin) that have an effect on bowel function. One of the classic responses to stress, for example, is rapid bowel emptying (diarrhoea). This was designed to make primitive man lighter when fleeing from dangerous predators.

Early research found that blood flow to the colon wall increased during stressful situations and emotional arousal, so that it looked more red. The amount of secretions increased, as did bowel movement. These were normal responses that did not seem to trigger any unpleasant symptoms, except for the expected diarrhoea.

Studies looking at small bowel function during stress suggest that people with I.B.S. have a more pronounced response than non-sufferers. In the normal small bowel, activity occurs in cycles depending on whether you have just eaten or have recently fasted. This pattern of activity followed by inactivity seems to be lost in some I.B.S. sufferers under stress so that bowel function becomes more irregular, especially during periods of fasting (e.g. overnight). During periods of active digestion, the number of contractions increases or decreases depending on the types of food eaten. Passage of some types of food through the small intestine is delayed, while transit of others is increased. This is not yet fully understood, but suggests that there is an underlying abnormality in gut movement in some people with I.B.S. There is also thought to be a link between anxiety and the likelihood of developing I.B.S. after a severe bout of gastroenteritis (*see page 9*). Other researchers have found that people with I.B.S. are more likely to have suffered from major emotional conflicts in childhood, particularly the loss of a parent or physical abuse – especially sexual abuse.

There is no doubt that some people with I.B.S. are under a lot of stress or are prone to anxiety. What is in doubt is whether this is cause or effect or whether it is totally unlinked. It is therefore worth looking at stress and how some of its symptoms can be overcome. If stress does make your symptoms worse, you can help yourself by addressing the stressful factors in your life and using relaxation techniques (*see Chapter 18*).

Candida yeast infection
Candida yeast infection is widely believed to be linked with symptoms of I.B.S. Many people find that dietary changes can reduce their symptoms. Candida is discussed further in Chapter 9.

Allergy, intolerance and trigger foods
There is no doubt that eating certain foods seems to trigger symptoms of I.B.S. in most sufferers, and that changing your diet can produce impressive results. Michelle Berriedale-Johnson has provided a variety of recipes in Chapters 11–16 to help make your dietary changes as easy and delicious as possible. Not all changes help all people, so introduce one change at a time for seven to ten days, then assess whether or not you find it beneficial. For further information, see Part Two: I.B.S. and Your Diet.

CHAPTER 3

Symptoms of I.B.S.

If you go and see your doctor about I.B.S., the chances are you will be prescribed drugs to help treat the symptoms. The main symptoms of I.B.S. are:

* Pain
* Distension or bloating
* Wind
* Constipation
* Diarrhoea
* Urgency (sudden urge to empty the bowels)
* Mucus production
* Incomplete bowel emptying
* Rectal pain
* Nausea

This chapter looks at these symptoms in more detail and provides information on the self-help measures, over-the-counter (OTC) medicines and prescribed drugs that are used to treat them.

Pain

The pain of I.B.S. is usually cramp-like or colicky, and comes and goes in waves. It can be felt anywhere in the abdomen but is often worse on the lower left-hand side – except in the form of I.B.S. known as Primary Foregut Motility Disorder, where bloating is more often linked with pain on the lower right-hand side of the abdomen. The pain may worsen after eating as this stimulates contraction of the colon – a phenomenon known as gastrocolic reflex – which is usually most pronounced in young infants who frequently fill their nappy after a meal. Sufferers usually find that opening the bowels or passing wind brings relief.

The abdominal pain experienced in I.B.S. seems to be a combination of stretch (distension pain) and spasm (constriction pain). Research has shown that by introducing a balloon into the bowel and periodically inflating it within the intestinal tract, from top to bottom, the pain and discomfort produced are similar to that experienced in I.B.S. This implies that distension may be the main factor causing the unpleasant discomfort that people with the condition experience.

When balloons are inflated at different sites in the colon, different people feel pain in different parts of the abdomen, so it is difficult to tell which part of the colon is in spasm in each sufferer. Just because pain is felt in the upper abdomen, for example, it doesn't mean the pain is coming from the underlying transverse part of the colon. Nerves from the gut pass back to the spinal cord and also supply other parts of the abdominal cavity on the way. This may lead to referred pain, in which pain coming from the bowel is interpreted by the brain as coming from the back, for example. This is the same principle as when pain from the heart (angina) is felt running down the left arm, or pain from the gallbladder is felt in the tip of the right shoulder.

If spasm occurs high in the gut, it can lead to nausea. Occurring lower down, it is more likely to cause constipation through slowing down and interfering with the passage of food through the colon, thus allowing more fluid to be absorbed.

Pain varies in a number of ways. It can help your doctor if you describe your pain as accurately as possible. Is it:

* Aching
* Burning
* Constant, intermittent or coming and going in waves
* Crushing
* Dragging
* Gnawing
* Throbbing
* Stabbing
* Stinging
* Superficial or deep
* Does it radiate to elsewhere in the body?

DO I NEED TO SEE A DOCTOR?

If the pain is moderate or short lived, lie down, rest and try cuddling a hot water bottle or taking a simple painkiller. Always read the label on the packaging of painkillers and never exceed the stated dose.

Call the doctor if the pain is unusually severe and you experience *any* of the following:

* Pain lasts more than 30 minutes
* Pain is accompanied by vomiting
* The abdomen becomes swollen or tender
* There is faintness, drowsiness or confusion
* There is a fever of 38 degrees or over
* You are pregnant or suspect you could be
* The pain has resulted from an accident or blow to the stomach

If you experience abdominal pain that keeps recurring or if your pain changes significantly, it is also important to see your doctor again. Sometimes other conditions causing abdominal pain can develop in someone with I.B.S., so any change in the nature of pain should always be reported. This is especially important if you also notice other related symptoms, such as a change in bowel habit or unexplained weight loss.

SIMPLE PAINKILLERS

So many painkillers are available over the counter that it can be difficult to know which to use. Some work better for certain types of ailment than others. Many new products contain a combination of ingredients for a broader range of pain relief. The following guide helps you mix and match your pain with the OTC remedy most likely to help. As with all medicines, always read the label on the packaging of painkillers and never exceed the stated dose. If you are unsure which painkiller you need, or are taking other medication, always ask your pharmacist for advice. For advice on complementary therapies (*see Chapter 18*).

Aspirin (acetylsalicylic acid)

Many people find that aspirin can improve mild to moderate abdominal pain associated with I.B.S. It works mainly by reducing the formation of inflammatory chemicals known as prostaglandins, and can damp down the swelling and stiffness of inflammation. It can also reduce a temperature through direct action on the brain. Aspirin is best taken in soluble, effervescent or enteric-coated forms to minimize stomach irritation.

Possible side-effects: stomach irritation (heartburn, feeling sick). Rarely: skin rashes, tightness in chest, intestinal bleeding.

It should not be used (except under medical supervision) by:

* Children under 12 years old
* Women who are pregnant or breastfeeding
* Those with a history of peptic ulcers, asthma, acute gout, kidney or liver problems or a blood-clotting disorder such as haemophilia
* Those taking other drugs – unless told by a pharmacist that there is no interaction

Paracetamol

Paracetamol is effective against mild to moderate pain that is not associated with inflammation and can be helpful for I.B.S. It works through a direct effect on the brain to kill pain and lower a fever. It does not reduce swelling or stiffness and does not irritate the stomach lining. If taking other over-the-counter remedies, make sure they do not also contain paracetamol or you could easily exceed the recommended dose. If in doubt, ask your pharmacist for advice.

Possible side-effects: liver damage if the dose is exceeded. Rarely: skin rash, blood disorders, pancreatitis.

It should not be used (except under medical supervision) by:

* Those with a high alcohol intake (increased risk of liver damage)
* Those with kidney or liver problems

Ibuprofen

Ibuprofen can also be helpful for relieving pain in I.B.S. Related to aspirin, it is classed as a non-steroidal anti-inflammatory drug (NSAID).

Possible side-effects: heartburn, nausea, diarrhoea. Rarely: skin rashes, wheezing, light-headedness, unusual bleeding or bruising.

It should not be used (except under medical supervision) by:

* Those with a history of peptic ulcers
* People with asthma
* Women who are pregnant or breastfeeding
* Those taking other drugs – unless told by a pharmacist that there is no interaction

Codeine

Codeine works on the nervous system to reduce the transmission of pain signals. It also changes the way pain is felt so, although it may still be there, it no longer seems to matter. Codeine is excellent for treating I.B.S. pain associated with diarrhoea and is often combined with other painkillers to help boost their effectiveness. It is best avoided if you are prone to constipation, however.

Possible side-effects: constipation, nausea, dizziness, drowsiness, sometimes vomiting. Should only be used occasionally as tolerance and even dependence may occur with long-term use.

It should not be used (except under medical supervision) by:

* Young children. Products vary depending on formulation. Some suggest use over the age of six years, others over the age of eight years

Dihydrocodeine

Dihydrocodeine is a more powerful version of codeine and is suitable for more severe pain associated with I.B.S. Until recently, it was available only on prescription, but a formulation combining dihydrocodeine with paracetamol is now available from pharmacists.

Possible side-effects: constipation, nausea, dizziness, drowsiness, sometimes vomiting. Should only be used occasionally as tolerance and even dependence is likely with long-term use.

It should not be used (except under medical supervision) by:

* Children under 12 years old

ANTISPASMODICS

Antispasmodic drugs act directly on the smooth muscle of the gut to prevent spasm. They are not successful in helping everyone with I.B.S. and can produce unwanted side-effects. These drugs should not be taken for undiagnosed abdominal pain or bloating (in case intestinal obstruction is present) and should not be taken during pregnancy or breastfeeding except under medical supervision.

Peppermint oil

Peppermint oil has a direct relaxant effect on the smooth muscle of the gut and helps to relieve pain, bloating, distension and wind. Capsules are taken 30 minutes before meals and may be used for up to three months. Do not break or chew capsules as it is important that the oil passes down to the large bowel to produce its medicinal effect.

Possible side-effects: may cause heartburn or a burning sensation around the anus, in which case, cut back on the dose.

Alverine citrate

Alverine citrate is an antispasmodic agent useful for treating smooth muscle spasm in both I.B.S. and painful periods. It comes in capsule form and is available over-the-counter or on prescription.

Possible side-effects: nausea, headache, itching, skin rashes or dizziness.

It should not be used (except under medical supervision):

- During pregnancy or breastfeeding

Mebeverine

Mebeverine has a direct action on the smooth muscle lining the gut to stop excessive contraction. This relieves spasm without affecting the normal activity of the gut. It relieves colicky abdominal pain, cramps, persistent non-specific diarrhoea (with or without alternating constipation) and flatulence. Mebeverine comes in the form of capsules, tablets or granules (with fibre), and is available over-the-counter or on prescription. It is taken three times a day, 20 minutes before meals. After a period of several weeks, when symptoms have improved, the dose can be slowly reduced.

Possible side-effects: no significant side-effects have been reported.

It should not be used (except under medical supervision):

- During pregnancy or breastfeeding
- By those with an inactive intestine (paralytic ileus), which can occur after abdominal surgery
- By those with an inherited metabolic condition known as porphyria

Dicyclomine

Dicyclomine (or dicycloverine) has a direct action on the smooth muscle lining the gut to stop excessive contraction. This reduces spasm without affecting the normal activity of the gut. It relieves colicky abdominal pain, cramps, persistent non-specific diarrhoea (with or without alternating constipation) and flatulence. Dicyclomine is available in the form of tablets, syrup or gel, usually on prescription, although the gel is available over-the-counter. It is normally taken three times a day, before or after meals.

Possible side-effects: dry mouth, thirst, dizziness, blurred vision, tiredness, drowsiness, rash, constipation, loss of appetite, nausea, headache or discomfort on urination.

It should not be used:

- By those with: glaucoma, myasthenia gravis, paralytic ileus, pyloric stenosis or an enlarged prostate gland

It is best avoided:

- By those with hiatus hernia associated with reflux oesophagitis (indigestion) as it may make symptoms worse

It should not be used (except under medical supervision):

- During pregnancy or breastfeeding
- By the elderly
- By sufferers of diarrhoea or ulcerative colitis
- If you have had a heart attack, heart failure or have high blood pressure
- If you suffer from hyperthyroidism
- If you have a fever

As there are so many people who should not take it, or should only do so with caution, dicyclomine is best taken under medical supervision only.

Propantheline

Propantheline is an antispasmodic agent useful for treating smooth muscle spasm and abdominal pain in I.B.S. It comes in tablet form and is available only on prescription. It is usually taken three times a day before meals and at bedtime.

Possible side-effects: dry mouth, blurred vision, dizziness, flushing, difficulty passing water, constipation. Rarely: skin rashes, fever or confusion.

For contraindications, see dicylomine, above.

Antidepressants

For patients who are resistant to treatment, a type of drug called a tri-cyclic antidepressant often produces good results. Although you are being treated with an antidepressant, it does not necessarily mean your doctor thinks you are depressed. The way in which these drugs work in I.B.S. is not fully understood. It may be that they increase the quantity of neurotransmitters (nerve communication chemicals) in nerve endings in the gut to reduce gut mobility and spasm, or to decrease pain perception. If your doctor prescribes an antidepressant tablet for you, ask how long you will need to take it and about possible side-effects.

Distension or bloating

Distension is often the most troublesome symptom of I.B.S. For some reason, distension seems to be worse in women than in men. It seems to be triggered by eating, and typically gets worse as the day progresses. Many women find they need to loosen tight clothing in the late afternoon and often tell embarrassed tales about being mistakenly congratulated for pregnancy.

Bloating seems to be associated with two of the three recently identified variants of I.B.S.: the spastic colon syndrome and primary motility disorder of the foregut. Several theories have been suggested to account for abdominal distension including:

- Excess abdominal gas.
- Flattening out (downward depression) of the diaphragm.
- Exaggerated spinal curve (lumbar lordosis).
- Fluid retention.
- Forward protrusion of the abdominal wall due to poor muscle tone.
- Excessive relaxation of the bowel, which is naturally constricted to form a tube around 2.85 metres long, although when fully relaxed it can more than double in length to 7 metres. It may well be that excessive and abnormal relaxation of the small intestines may occur throughout the day, lengthening the gut so that it occupies more space, leading to abdominal distension.

Unfortunately, there is no real orthodox medical treatment for bloating and distension but many herbal remedies can help (*see Chapter 18*).

Wind

Wind (flatus) is a common symptom in I.B.S. Excessive flatulence often accompanies abdominal pain and bloating. It burbles around causing pain, distension and embarrassing noises (borborygmi) until escaping – upwards through the mouth or downwards through the anus – suddenly and sometimes explosively. In general, wind in the stomach is expelled upwards by burping, while wind in the small intestines and colon is expelled via the anus. Bowel gases come from several different sources:

* Gas present in fizzy drinks
* Air swallowed with food
* Air swallowed nervously by some people (aerophagia)
* Gases released during bacterial fermentation of fibre in the large bowel

It used to be thought that air swallowed naturally during eating and drinking was the cause of the problem. This is not the case, however, as analysis of the gas shows that only a small fraction of intestinal gas comes from the atmosphere.

Most intestinal gas comes from colonic bacteria breaking down indigestible fibre and starches not absorbed in the small intestine. They do this through a process of fermentation that releases short chain fatty acids, heat and gases such as hydrogen, carbon dioxide, methane and sometimes foul-smelling sulphur-containing gases such as hydrogen sulphide. This excess gas cannot be reabsorbed to any great extent, although some passes into the bloodstream and is excreted through the lungs. A small amount is used up in other bacterial metabolic reactions, but around 1–2.5 litres per day is expelled through the rectum.

Surprisingly, there is no evidence that people with I.B.S. produce more intestinal gas than people without symptoms. Research suggests that most people pass gas 12–20 times per day. Similarly, the make-up of flatus gases is no different in people with I.B.S. than in others, and the amount of gas remaining in the bowels at any one time is similar (up to 200 ml). Some differences have been noticed, however. Wind passes through the gut of people with I.B.S. more slowly than in those without symptoms, and sufferers seem to be more sensitive to the distension it causes. The gas is also more likely to pass backwards through the bowel and to reflux up into the stomach to be expelled by burping. Wind symptoms therefore seem to be due to abnormal movement of the intestines and disordered passage of wind through the gut, rather than to the production of excess gas.

Some people with excessive wind lack the right enzymes to digest certain foods, especially dairy foods, which require enzymes such as lactase to break down milk sugar (lactose). Inadequate amounts of lactase lead to lactose intolerance, which can produce wind and loose bowels. These people will find their symptoms improve dramatically on cutting out milk-based products from their diet (*see Chapter 10*).

Some foods contain compounds that increase gas production in everyone. Beans, for example, contain substances such as raffinose. Soaking beans overnight before cooking will help to aid their digestion and decrease flatulence.

If you are prone to excessive wind:

- Eat meals slowly, chewing each mouthful thoroughly
- Avoid food or drinks that are too hot
- Avoid fizzy drinks such as cola or champagne
- Avoid chewing gum or sucking boiled sweets
- Try drinking herbal teas containing chamomile, fennel, ginger, sage or peppermint
- Avoid foods that promote bacterial fermentation and gas production such as: beans, lentils, cauliflower, cabbage, broccoli, Brussels sprouts, celery, onions, carrots, raisins, bananas, apricots, wheatgerm, cucumber, milk and milk products

Orthodox medical treatment for wind includes:

- Peppermint oil capsules *(see page 24)*
- Charcoal tablets or biscuits which absorb unpleasant flatus odours and excess gas
- Supplements containing simethicone (activated dimethicone), which are available in chemists

Constipation

Constipation is usually defined as passing bowel motions less than twice a week, or straining at stool for more than a quarter of the time. Constipation is a common and distressing feature of I.B.S. and occurs more often than diarrhoea. It is made worse by uncoordinated contractions and spasm of the muscular bowel walls, which squash bowel contents rather than pushing them through. As a result, the bowels may not open for days at a time – so-called slow transit constipation. When they do, straining is necessary to push out hard pellets resembling rabbit droppings, or thin ribbons of faeces. Because bowel contents stay inside you for longer than usual, increased amounts of fluid are reabsorbed from them. This makes the faeces harder in consistency, and they may scratch the anal margin to cause blood staining after voiding.

Laxatives

Laxatives fall into four main groups depending on how they work:

1 Bulking agents (mild)
2 Faecal softeners (mild)
3 Stimulants (moderate irritant action)
4 Osmotic agents (lactulose is gentle; some salts have a strong action)

The overall effect of laxatives is to increase the fluid content of bowel motions, increase intestinal movement and, in some cases, to alter the way in which the colon contracts.

Six out of ten users take a stimulant laxative that works by irritating the colon and may make symptoms of I.B.S. worse.

Unfortunately, prolonged use of a laxative will trigger insensitivity to that laxative so more and more has to be taken to achieve the same effect. When the laxative is stopped, rebound constipation can occur. If constipation lasts more than a few days while taking a laxative, check with your doctor before continuing to use the treatment.

Laxatives can help when used wisely. As a general rule:

* Do not use in the presence of undiagnosed abdominal pain, nausea or vomiting
* Only take them when absolutely necessary and do not mix them
* Do not use during pregnancy or while breastfeeding, except under medical supervision
* Use the mildest one to cope with your symptoms – if in doubt, consult a pharmacist
* A bulking agent (e.g. fibre supplements) or gentle osmotic laxative (e.g. lactulose) is a good first-line agent to try
* Stimulant laxatives such as senna should be avoided as much as possible
* Rectal preparations (suppositories, microenemas) are often as helpful as – or better than – taking oral laxatives and less likely to cause side-effects
* Do not exceed the stated dose
* Drink plenty of fluids and increase the amount of fibre in your diet
* Take regular exercise
* Try abdominal massage to encourage peristalsis and bowel emptying
* Taking a tablespoon or two of cold-pressed oils such as virgin olive oil, safflower, walnut or sesame, can help to get constipated motions moving

---

Bulking agents

Bulking agents contain indigestible plant fibre that is taken with water or sprinkled onto food. They increase the volume of bowel motions by absorbing water, softening the faeces and helping bowel walls get a better grip for propelling motions downwards. They work very well, but it is important to drink plenty of water. Some people find them unpalatable, and the added fibre may cause flatulence and bloating, making I.B.S. symptoms worse. Don't keep taking the same sort of fibre product month after month as its effectiveness will decrease and your symptoms may return as your bowel bacteria adapt to it. Keep varying the types of fibre that you eat (*see Chapter 7*). The following bulking agents can be obtained from health-food stores:

- Natural bran – introduce at a dose of 1 tablespoon two to three times a day with meals and vary according to response
- Wheat husks
- Ispaghula husks
- Sterculia
- Methyl cellulose
- Psyllium

The onset of action is slow and gentle: usually 12–24 hours, but it may take several days. You will need to persist with treatment for a week or two before you establish a regular bowel pattern.

Bulking agents should not be used by people with undiagnosed abdominal pain or vomiting in case a degree of bowel obstruction is present.

People with functional diarrhoea (*see page 7*) may also find bulking agents useful to absorb excess fluid.

Faecal softeners

Faecal softeners work by increasing the penetration of water and fats into solid bowel motions. This softens them, eases straining and is useful for painful conditions such as anal fissure, haemorrhoids, proctitis, and where straining should be avoided. The onset of action takes 24–48 hours.

LIQUID PARAFFIN EMULSION

This has a lubricating action which works by softening faeces and easing their passage. Hardly any is absorbed from the gut and it is relatively safe, although some people find it unpleasant to take. Available over-the-counter or on prescription, 10–30 ml should be taken at night when required, although not immediately before going to bed. The use of liquid paraffin emulsion should be restricted to temporary relief of constipation. Repeated use is not advisable as it can affect the absorption of vitamins and minerals in the gut, and may seep through the anus causing irritation and embarrassing moistness. There is a possible risk of respiratory inhalation in debilitated patients that may lead to pneumonia.

DOCUSATE SODIUM

This has a detergent action which reduces the surface tension of bowel motions and encourages softening through water absorption. It also stimulates the secretion of water and salts into the gut, and can therefore be classified as a stimulant laxative, too. It is available over-the-counter or on prescription in the form of capsules, oral solution and enemas. Treatment is usually started with larger doses (up to 50 ml per day in divided doses), which are decreased as symptoms improve. Docusate sodium may cause an unpleasant aftertaste or burning sensation in the mouth. This can be minimized by drinking plenty of water after taking the solution.

Stimulant laxatives

Stimulant laxatives work by irritating the bowel wall and increasing the movement of the colon. Some purge the bowel and can cause a sudden, violent action of watery motions with intestinal cramps and griping. This will obviously make I.B.S. symptoms worse. These laxatives should only be used on specific occasions and are best avoided by most people with I.B.S. If used regularly, their effectiveness will be reduced as the bowel becomes used to them – and when you stop taking them, rebound constipation can occur. In the long term, they may even trigger a more serious condition known as a non-functioning colon, in which the colon stops working.

Once taken, the onset of action is usually rapid – within 6–12 hours. Stimulant laxatives should not be used by people with undiagnosed abdominal pain or vomiting in case a degree of bowel obstruction is present. They may also affect the body's salt balance.

Senna is the gentlest stimulant laxative in this group (*see below*). Cascara and castor oil are powerful stimulant laxatives whose use is now virtually obsolete and not recommended for people with I.B.S.

Bisacodyl

The tablets are usually taken at night and work within 10–12 hours, although they may cause griping abdominal pains (colic). The suppositories are usually inserted in the morning and work within 20–60 minutes. However, local irritation may occur. Both tablets and suppositories are available over-the-counter or on prescription.

Senna

Derived from the seed pods of the plant *Senna alexandrina*, senna is a powerful laxative, available over-the-counter. Usually taken at night starting with a low dose, it acts within 8–12 hours. Reserve senna for occasional use only – it is not recommended as a long-term treatment as it may trigger bowel cramps and make symptoms of I.B.S. worse.

Phenolphthalein

A constituent of many over-the-counter laxative preparations, phenolphthalein may cause rashes in some people and may colour alkaline urine pink.

Osmotic laxatives

Osmotic laxatives work by drawing fluid into the bowels to soften stools and provide lubrication to ease constipation. They should always be taken with plenty of water. Salts of sodium, potassium or magnesium have a powerful action and are also known as saline purges. Their onset of action is rapid – within 1–4 hours in some cases – and can verge on the violent or incontinent. Lactulose is one of the gentle members of this group, usually working within 24–48 hours of the first dose.

LACTULOSE/LACTITOL

Lactulose is a synthetic double sugar (disaccharide) that is not digested or absorbed from the small intestine. It has an osmotic effect which draws water into the bowel and interferes with fluid absorption. Once in the large bowel, lactulose is digested by normal colonic bacteria, which convert it into short-chain organic acids. This encourages bacterial growth, bulks up the size of the stool and raises stool acidity. These actions encourage peristalsis and help to move moist faeces through the colon. It is available as a liquid or dry powder which some people find unpalatable as it is quite sweet. Lactulose can be used safely by most people, including pregnant or breastfeeding women, the elderly, diabetics and children over the age of five.

MAGNESIUM SALTS

This treatment is useful when rapid emptying of the bowel is needed (such as before a bowel investigation) and for some people with an abnormally slow bowel transit time. However, it should be used only occasionally as it may cause colic. Magnesium salts should not be used by those with poor kidney or liver function, except under medical supervision.

SODIUM SALTS

These are mainly used rectally as microenemas. They are not recommended to be taken by mouth as they may cause salt and water retention in some people. Sodium salts should not be taken by people with high blood pressure or heart or kidney problems, except under medical supervision.

Diarrhoea

Diarrhoea is usually defined as a loose consistency of stool plus increased frequency of bowel motions that lasts longer than two weeks. Your doctor will want to know:

* How long you've had it
* Whether the stools are watery or just soft

- If they're sloppy or like porridge
- If there are any formed stools
- Their colour
- If you have noticed any blood, pus or slime mixed in with them
- Whether you have feelings of urgency to open your bowels
- Whether there is any sensation of incomplete evacuation
- Whether you have to get up at night to evacuate your bowel
- Whether the motions float or are difficult to flush away

I.B.S. is probably the commonest cause of persistent diarrhoea. It occurs when the bowel works overtime to secrete increased amounts of mucus and to hasten the intestinal contents through. The problem is usually intermittent in nature and associated with other classic symptoms such as distension, bloating, excess wind and sensations of incomplete bowel movement. The diarrhoea associated with I.B.S. is often worse in the early hours of the morning, between 5 and 10 a.m. (morning rush syndrome). In this case, an anti-diarrhoeal drug such as loperamide will help if taken last thing at night and after the first bowel action every morning. Treatment should only be used for short periods without consulting your doctor.

If your bowels are very loose, it is also worth avoiding fruit juices and prunes and cutting down on milk and other dairy products. Drink plenty of fluids to counter dehydration, especially if you are only passing small amounts of dark urine. Fibre supplements will also help by bulking up bowel contents and absorbing excess fluid, but may take a few days to work. If diarrhoea lasts more than a few days, check with your doctor before continuing to use an anti-diarrhoeal treatment. Diarrhoea that lasts longer than two weeks should always be investigated to find out its cause.

ANTI-DIARRHOEAL DRUGS

Drugs to stop diarrhoea are mainly synthetic opiates, some of which (e.g. codeine) are metabolized to morphine in the body. These drugs interact with opiate receptors in the bowel to regulate smooth muscle tone and slow bowel transit time. They are useful for treating I.B.S. symptoms in some people, especially those with Functional Diarrhoea Syndrome.

Codeine phosphate

Codeine phosphate acts as both an anti-diarrhoea agent and a moderately strong painkiller. It is useful in I.B.S. when diarrhoea is accompanied by colicky pain – but only if the diagnosis of I.B.S. has been medically confirmed.

Loperamide

Loperamide is a synthetic opiate but is poorly absorbed and does not affect the central nervous system to cause drowsiness. It is the most popular drug for helping to treat diarrhoea and urgency in I.B.S. Possible side-effects include abdominal cramps, skin rashes, impaired bowel function (paralytic ileus) and bloating. If pregnant or breast-feeding, only take under medical supervision.

Co-phenotrope

A mixture of diphenoxylate hydrochloride (related to pethidine) and atropine sulphate, co-phenotrope works by slowing bowel movement and reducing fluid secretion into the gut. It is usually taken every six hours until symptoms subside. Possible side-effects include allergic reactions, dry mouth, blurred vision, dizziness and nausea.

Urgency

Urgency is the sudden need to rush to the toilet to open your bowels. This may herald a bout of diarrhoea or an attack of rectal spasm and pain. Some sufferers, especially those with Functional Diarrhoea Syndrome (*see page 7*), are unable to travel far from home because of the speed with which they need to open their bowels. This symptom is usually made worse by following a high-fibre diet, but may respond to treatment with anti-diarrhoeal drugs such as loperamide or Imodium.

Mucus production

Increased production of mucus is triggered by mechanical stimulation of mucus glands in the lining of the colon. It is mainly associated with the spastic colon form of I.B.S. in which disordered contraction and movement in the colon keeps bulky, dry faeces in contact with the bowel wall for longer than normal. Occasionally, excess mucus production is a sign of a mucus-producing polyp, inflammation or infection. If mucus production is a new symptom for you, and one your doctor doesn't know about, tell him or her during your next consultation.

Incomplete bowel emptying

Many sufferers notice an unpleasant sensation of not completely evacuating the bowels after voiding. This seems to be due to over-sensitivity of the rectum so that it continues to feel as if there is unfinished business to attend to. This may keep you on the toilet for long periods of time, and may encourage you to strain. Straining can lead to unpleasant rectal spasm (tenesmus) and rectal pain that can take your breath away and make you feel faint (*see below*). You can reduce the pressure of straining by rocking forwards on your hips so that you are leaning over your knees while sitting on the toilet bowl.

Rectal pain

Rectal pain affects most people at some time in their life. Also known as rectal angina or proctalgia fugax, it is a severe pain felt deep in the rectum. While not usually associated with any particular condition, it can occur in people with I.B.S. It is more common in men than women and often occurs at night. It is sometimes brought on by straining, constipation or passing wind, and can also be caused by vigorous exercise when the bowel is full. The spasm tends to last from 1–15 minutes and then subsides on its own. Occasionally, it may last as long as an hour. The next bowel motion passed may take the form of a thin ribbon through having been squeezed and compressed by the cramping lower bowel and rectum.

This is not a diagnosis that should be made without medical assessment – always seek medical advice for recurrent pain. Researchers believe this condition is due to spasm of the pelvic floor muscles. Eating or drinking may bring relief, as may applying pressure to the perineum (the area in front of the anus). You can do this, for example, by sitting astride the edge of your bath. Some people find inserting a suppository relieves the spasm. If attacks are severe and recurrent, your GP may prescribe glyceryl trinitrate (sublingual tablets or spray), which often brings prompt relief – although treatment may be followed by a rebound headache. The good news is that attacks are rare over the age of 50.

Nausea

Nausea is not experienced by all people with I.B.S. It seems to be linked with spasm of the small intestine rather than the large bowel, and may occur in the primary foregut motility disorder variant of I.B.S. (*see page 7*). It may be brought on by backward passage of wind (reflux) through the intestines. If you suffer from recurrent nausea or vomiting, you should always tell your doctor.

Other symptoms associated with I.B.S.

Research shows that people with I.B.S. are more likely to suffer from heartburn, indigestion, flushing, palpitations, migraine and urinary symptoms throughout life than those without I.B.S. Sufferers are also more likely to develop asthma. In one study, 22.4 per cent of people with I.B.S. had over-sensitive lung airways compared with 12.2 per cent of those without I.B.S. This suggests that I.B.S. may be linked to a smooth muscle or nervous system disorder which affects the nerves or smooth muscle fibres found in both the lungs and gut.

Other symptoms that commonly occur in people with I.B.S. include:

* Tiredness
* Lack of energy
* Acid reflux into the mouth
* Mild weight loss
* Recurrent back pain
* Recurrent loin pain

- Painful sexual intercourse
- Chest pain
- Shortness of breath on exercise and wheeziness
- Hyperventilation (overbreathing)

These symptoms are common – up to 80 per cent of people with I.B.S. also have indigestion or heartburn, for example. This may well result from disordered contraction and movement throughout the length of the gut.

All these findings indicate that I.B.S. is only part of a spectrum of symptoms to which certain people are prone. They may have:

- A more active nervous system
- Increased contractility of smooth muscles, including those in the gut
- Increased levels of circulating chemicals that cause constriction or dilation of nerves or muscles (vaso-active peptides)

It may be that some people are born with a natural predisposition to I.B.S., and that symptoms start only when they are exposed to a trigger factor. Researchers have found that people with I.B.S. are more likely to have suffered from abdominal pain in childhood for example – perhaps triggered by a viral illness. These recurrent attacks are often dismissed as growing pains and are eventually forgotten by parents. One study claims that as many as one in six older children have symptoms of I.B.S., which may be bad enough to restrict their lifestyle. A questionnaire given to 851 school children found that boys and girls were equally affected and that 16 per cent had one or more symptoms of:

- Abdominal pain
- Altered bowel habit
- Urgency
- Incomplete evacuation of the bowels

The symptoms of I.B.S. are often similar to those of other gut problems, including inflammatory bowel disease and bowel cancer. As a general rule, if your bowel symptoms develop for the first time when you are over the age of 45, your doctor will want to investigate further to rule out other more potentially serious bowel problems. If your symptoms are due to a tumour, for example, you have a good chance of being cured if you bring them to the attention of a doctor at an early, treatable stage. For this reason, irritable bowel syndrome is not a condition that anyone should diagnose themselves.

Is there a cure?

Despite active research, the exact cause of I.B.S. remains unknown, and therefore a cure is still elusive. Many people with I.B.S. find their symptoms improve with time and disappear in later life. One study found that after five years, 70 per cent of sufferers were free of symptoms. As a result, it is rare to see an elderly person with I.B.S.

Dietary and lifestyle changes can help to relieve symptoms in many cases, and food supplements or, if necessary, medications, are often helpful in controlling bothersome symptoms such as recurrent diarrhoea or constipation. There is no need to wait until you reach your 70s to gain relief from this unpleasant condition. Part Two of this book looks at how changing your diet can improve your symptoms, and there are over 60 recipes in Part Three. Further lifestyle changes and food supplements are examined in Part Four.

Always tell a doctor as soon as possible if you notice:

* A change in your usual bowel habit
* Any blood or blackness in your stools
* Any unexplained weight loss
* Bowel symptoms for the first time if you are over 45

CHAPTER 4

Diagnosing I.B.S.

Unfortunately, there are no tests for I.B.S. that can definitely confirm you have the condition. Because so many other bowel problems produce similar symptoms, any investigations you have are intended to rule out other conditions such as ulcerative colitis, Crohn's disease, diverticular disease and bowel cancer.

Originally, I.B.S. was looked on as a diagnosis of exclusion – it was only diagnosed once other more serious bowel problems were ruled out. This view is now less common as, for most people, it would lead to many unnecessary and at times unpleasant investigations. Instead, careful questioning is used more and more to diagnose I.B.S. on clinical grounds according to the Rome Criteria (*see page 2*), although investigations are often needed to rule out other conditions such as those mentioned above.

You may have some of the following investigations during evaluation of your bowel symptoms, but it is rare to have them all. As a routine, most people with symptoms suggestive of I.B.S. are likely to have some basic blood screening tests and a sigmoidoscopy (*see below*). If you are aged over 40, or have lost weight recently, you will probably have further investigations such as a barium enema or colonoscopy (*see below*). If you are suffering from diarrhoea, a small biopsy of your bowel wall may be taken (e.g. during sigmoidoscopy) for microscopic examination to rule out inflammatory bowel disease. You may also have a lactose intolerance test and a biopsy of the small intestine if lactase deficiency is thought to be a diagnostic possibility.

In pure I.B.S., all tests should produce normal results. Unfortunately, being told by a specialist that all the tests are negative, or that 'nothing is wrong with you' is upsetting – until you realize that the doctor isn't trying to say you are imagining your symptoms, but that nothing potentially serious or life-threatening is present. This reassurance that symptoms are due to I.B.S. means that different treatments – drugs or self-help regimes – can be tried to see which suits you best, with no fear that another diagnosis requiring a different treatment has been missed.

Abdominal examination

Abdominal examination (palpation) is essential to look for signs of tenderness, fullness or obvious masses. In cases of I.B.S., this examination does not usually find anything abnormal, although some patients will have a boggy colon (known as the squelch sign) and the last part of the colon (sigmoid colon) may be loaded with faeces and tender. This tenderness may be found down the lower left-hand side of your abdomen (descending and sigmoid colon) or on the right (position of ascending colon).

Rectal examination

A digital rectal examination is important for anyone with a bowel problem. This is only slightly uncomfortable and gives important information regarding the texture of the bowel lining, whether the rectum is full or empty of stool, and can enable the detection of rectal tumours as 75 per cent are within reach of the examining finger.

This procedure is nowhere near as unpleasant as most people think but can be uncomfortable rather than painful. Most patients describe the sensation as similar to that experienced when constipated. The doctor uses a colourless, water-based jelly as a lubricant. Only the index finger is inserted – which, if you think about it, is much thinner than the width of the average bowel motion.

In cases of I.B.S., the results of the digital rectal examination will be entirely normal, although the lining of the rectum may seem loose in some people.

Blood tests

Most people with symptoms of I.B.S. will have routine blood tests performed to help rule out problems such as anaemia, infection or an underactive thyroid gland. If you have diarrhoea, the salt balance of your body will also be measured to make sure you have not developed a low potassium level due to excessive fluid loss.

If coeliac disease is suspected, you may be offered a special blood allergy test to detect antibodies against gliadin, the small protein (polypeptide) found in gluten to which sufferers are sensitive (*see Chapter 6*).

Stool culture

If you have prolonged or recurrent diarrhoea, your stools will usually be cultured to look for signs of infective bacteria, viruses or other parasites. This is especially important if you have recently travelled abroad, if other members of your family are affected or if your occupation involves food handling. You will need to provide a fresh stool sample, preferably sent to the hospital while it is still steaming, to increase the chances of any pathogens being found. It will take a few days for the stools to be cultured and the results to become available.

Faecal occult bloods

In this test, a small stool sample is smeared onto a special reagent paper containing a chemical (e.g. the gum, guaiac) that reacts with hidden (occult) blood and changes colour when activated by a developer. This test is a routine screen for early bowel cancer but false positives are common – especially if you have cleaned your teeth vigorously the night before, recently eaten red meat or have piles. If the test comes back positive, there is usually no cause for concern – it will be repeated two or three times before any decision to investigate further is taken.

Plain abdominal x-ray

A plain abdominal x-ray is not usually very helpful, but is sometimes requested to rule out abnormal collections of fluid or air in the abdominal cavity. It is often performed at the beginning of a barium enema to provide images for comparison with those obtained during the procedure.

Ultrasound

During this investigation, which is simple and painless, a special probe is run up and down the outside of your abdomen to pass high-frequency, inaudible sound waves through your body. This is the same test used during pregnancy to check the development of a growing baby. The ultrasound waves bounce back off tissue planes and collections of fluid or air to give a pattern that is interpreted by a computer to form an image. Ultrasound is best carried out while you have a full bladder to help orientate the images produced.

Proctoscopy

This involves visually examining the inner walls of the rectum. A small, lubricated speculum is inserted to expose the walls. This helps the doctor see if the rectum is inflamed, bleeding, has internal piles or other lesions. In cases of pure I.B.S., a proctoscopy will show perfectly normal and healthy looking tissues.

Sigmoidoscopy

A sigmoidoscope is used to view the inner walls of the lower (sigmoid) part of the colon. There are two sorts of sigmoidoscope – rigid and flexible. The rigid sigmoidoscope is a narrow instrument around 30 cm (12 inches) long with illumination at the end. It has several channels along it through which the surgeon can pass air, or a special instrument to take a biopsy. The rigid sigmoidoscope lets the doctor examine your bowel lining up to around 20 cm (8 inches) of the anus. The flexible sigmoidoscope can pass further up and allows 60 cm (24 inches) of the lower bowel to be visually inspected using fibre optics.

During either procedure, you will be asked to lie on your left side, with your knees drawn up slightly. After gently inserting the narrow end of the instrument into the lower rectum, air is pumped into your bowel to gently spread the walls apart away from the advancing tip of the instrument. As this air escapes, it may produce noises similar to flatus and many patients are embarrassed by it. Remember though – it's not your wind causing the problem, but that pumped in by the doctor. No-one else in the room will think anything of it, so try not to be upset. During the procedure, the doctor will assess the appearance (colour, granularity, sheen) of the bowel lining (mucosa) and look for any obvious inflammation, bleeding sites, masses or polyps. He or she will also note how strongly and frequently your lower bowel contracts when the instrument is advanced. If contractions are powerful – known as the winging sign – it is a good indication that the type of I.B.S. associated with constipation, rectal distension and abdominal pain (spastic colon syndrome) is present. It implies that you should take all possible steps to avoid constipation and rectal distension in the future as this will go a long way to controlling your symptoms.

The air pumped into your bowel may also cause distension pain similar to your usual I.B.S. symptoms. If this happens, it is important to tell the doctor – again, this is a good sign that your symptoms are related to muscular activity within the bowel rather than to any other disease process.

Some of the wind pumped into your bowel may remain inside for a day or so afterwards, causing distension, discomfort and flatus, although most patients have few problems.

Colonoscopy

Colonoscopy uses a longer, flexible instrument than the sigmoido-scope, to inspect further up the colon, usually under light sedation. You will be given a powerful laxative (or oral bowel cleansing solution) to take beforehand, which acts within 10–14 hours. This helps to empty the bowel and provide better views for the doctor.

Colonoscopy is usually only performed if a change in bowel habit such as constipation or diarrhoea is accompanied by persistent bleeding or weight loss, or if there is a family history of inheritable bowel problems. It is more accurate than a barium enema but is limited by its poor ability to reach the first part of the colon (caecum). People aged 40–50 years are often investigated routinely (as bowel tumours have to be considered), but the percentage of abnormal findings picked up is low.

Barium enema

Soft tissues such as the bowel do not show up very well on x-ray. One way to examine your bowel is to coat its internal lining with a substance that shows up on x-ray, such as barium sulphate. Before having a barium enema, you will be asked not to eat anything the night before, and to drink plenty of fluids instead. You will also be given a powerful laxative to empty your bowel so that faeces don't get in the way of the test.

The test will take place in the hospital radiology department. A tube is gently inserted into your rectum, and a small amount of barium mixture pumped in along with some air to provide a good contrast on the x-ray. During the procedure, you will be asked to lie on a special table that allows your body to be tilted up and down at different angles. This lets gravity do the work of spreading the barium solution to coat your inner bowel walls. The radiologist will watch views of your bowel the whole time, and print radiographs at certain points, especially if anything unusual such as an ulcer or solid mass shows up. While a barium enema usually provides good views of the first part of the colon (caecum), any faeces that remain stuck to the bowel walls will interfere with the results. They can show up as solids that may be misinterpreted as a polyp or tumour requiring subsequent colonoscopy for further inspection. The overall accuracy of a barium enema is therefore usually quoted as around 85 per cent.

Having a barium enema is not the most pleasant test in the world, and can be uncomfortable, noisy and messy. It is not usually painful, however. Afterwards, the solution will be passed as a runny bowel motion. You may pass wind and white, lumpy bowel motions over the next few days.

Transit bowel studies

Some people with severe constipation may be offered transit studies to see how fast bowel contents move through the gut. You will be given a special substance to swallow that gives off safe amounts of radioisotopes or other markers that can be accurately measured. If, 96 hours later, 20 per cent or more of these markers have not been voided, and are still detectable in your gut, this shows that the transit of bowel contents is sluggish.

Bowel pressure studies

Abnormality of bowel contractions (motility) can be mapped out using small tubes containing pressure sensors. These are placed in the intestines and record motility changes, which can be relayed to show pressure changes occurring throughout a 24-hour period.

Lactose tolerance tests

If lactose intolerance is suspected, you may have tests to check for this. For further information, *see Chapter 6*.

Gluten tolerance tests

If gluten intolerance is suspected, you may have tests to check for this. For further information, *see Chapter 6*.

Computed tomography (CT scan)

A CT scan is not often performed during investigations of I.B.S. unless there is a suggestion of a mass in the abdomen. This is because the procedure is expensive and exposes you to radiation, so is only performed where it is likely to provide some significant benefit. CT scans involve taking multiple x-ray views across your body at different angles, which are then interpreted by computer to produce a cross-sectional image (slice) at various levels.

Magnetic resonance imaging (MRI)

MRI does not involve the use of x-rays and is therefore preferable to a CT scan if this type of procedure is indicated. It uses a strong magnetic field to align the molecules in your body. A pulse of radio waves is then passed through you to knock the molecules slightly out of alignment. As the molecules bounce back into place, they give out a weak radio signal, which is picked up and interpreted by a computer. This gives an excellent cross-sectional or three-dimensional image of different parts of your body without any known risks or side-effects. The procedure is expensive, however, and is not routinely used when investigating I.B.S.

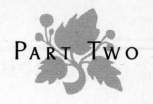

PART TWO

I.B.S. and Diet

CHAPTER 5

Eat to beat I.B.S.

I.B.S. is virtually unheard of in countries where a healthy high-fibre, wholefood diet is followed. The sort of food we eat in the West, and some of the nutritional deficiencies we may suffer as a result, may play a major part in triggering symptoms. Although this is not fully understood, making dietary changes to include some foods and avoid others helps to improve symptoms in most people with I.B.S.

Foods that most consistently worsen symptoms of I.B.S. include:

Milk and dairy products such as cheese (but rarely yoghurt)
Wheat, gluten and wheat bran
Oats, rye and barley
Yeast
Chocolate
Fatty foods
Potatoes
Citrus fruits (e.g. oranges, grapefruit)
Tea and coffee
Salads, tomatoes, pulses and cabbage
Onions and garlic
Eggs
Meat
Acidic foods (e.g. vinegar)
Artificial sweeteners
Artificial additives
Very spicy foods

If you suspect one or more of these foods is causing your symptoms, try eating the food(s) for one week, then cut them out the next to see if your symptoms change.

As a general rule, if you suffer from:

Constipation Follow a high-fibre diet.
Constipation plus bloating and wind Follow a low-fibre diet and take a bulking agent such as psyllium.
Diarrhoea Try following a low-fibre diet initially, and if this doesn't improve symptoms, try the Addenbrooke's exclusion diet (*see page 64*).

Where possible, eat meals that are as pure as possible:

- Wheat-free
- Gluten-free
- Lactose-free
- Yeast-free
- Not genetically modified (GM)

The delicious recipes by Michelle Berriedale-Johnson in Part Three of this book will make this easy for you.

Eating patterns

How you eat can also play a role in improving symptoms. Eat little and often to keep your blood sugar levels up – never skip a meal, especially breakfast. Try eating several small meals spread throughout the day rather than the traditional three large meals with little in-between. If your lifestyle makes eating three daily meals necessary, then follow the old advice: breakfast like a king, lunch like a lord and dine like a pauper.

Eat meals in an unrushed fashion – leave plenty of time to eat so you don't bolt down your food and swallow excessive amounts of air. It will also help to sit down at a table to eat rather than grabbing a snack on the move, which is more likely to be bolted down and inadequately chewed.

Eliminating suspect food groups

Try avoiding certain groups of products for a week or two at a time to see if symptoms improve, then reintroduce them to see if symptoms worsen again. This can help identify whether or not your symptoms are related to dairy products, wheat, fibre etc. More detailed information on elimination diets can be found in the next chapter.

* Avoid dairy products altogether for one week to see if your symptoms change, as some people diagnosed as having I.B.S. may have lactose intolerance instead – difficulty in absorbing a sugar, lactose, found in milk *(see page 83)*. While avoiding dairy products or restricting your diet in any way, take a good vitamin and mineral supplement containing calcium. If your symptoms do improve, ask your doctor whether you need investigations for lactose intolerance. Also request dietary advice from a nutritionist to ensure you are not at risk of becoming deficient in calcium or other nutrients from cutting out dairy foods over a longer period.
* Cut back on your intake of red meat for at least one week to see if this improves your symptoms. Eat more fish and skinless white meat in its place.
* Some people with I.B.S. are sensitive to acidic foods such as oranges, grapefruit, tomatoes and vinegar. Again, try cutting them out to see if this helps.
* Some people find that spicy food irritates their bowel lining and makes symptoms worse. Try eating lots of spicy foods one week, then cutting them out the next to see if your symptoms change.

Tips for improving your diet

* Try increasing your intake of fibre slowly. If bran seems to make your symptoms worse – even after persevering with it for two or three weeks – concentrate on getting fibre from vegetables, rice and fruit.

* Instead of bran, you could try a supplement containing ispaghula, psyllium or sterculia. Be sure to alternate these supplements – if you take them all at once you will lose the benefits *(see Chapter 17)*.

* If a high-fibre diet seems to make your symptoms worse, then try a low-fibre diet for a week or so to see if this helps – but drink plenty of fluids to reduce the risk of worsening constipation.

* Eat more fresh fruit and vegetables – especially nuts, seeds, figs, apricots, prunes, peas and beans.

* Eat more fish, especially oily fish.

* Eat more complex, unrefined carbohydrates such as wholegrain bread, wholemeal pasta, brown rice and unsweetened wholegrain breakfast cereals such as muesli or porridge (assuming that your symptoms are not made worse by wheat).

* Try adding live bio yoghurt (containing a culture of Lactobacilli) to your diet. Many sufferers find this relieves their symptoms. Lactobacilli have been shown to survive stomach acids and can colonize the bowel with healthy bacteria.

* Drink more fluids, especially bottled water or herbal teas. Aim to drink 2–3 litres of fluid per day.

* Limit your intake of artificial sweeteners and additives (E numbers), as some people find these aggravate symptoms.

* Cut back on sugar and salt and processed or convenience foods.

* Cut down on the amount of saturated fat in your diet. Avoid full-fat dairy products such as butter, cream and whole milk. Instead, try semi-skimmed or skimmed milk and spreads made from olive oil. Low-fat fromage frais is a delicious and healthy substitute for cream.

* Don't fry or roast your food – grill, bake, casserole or steam instead.

* If wind is a problem, avoid beans, cabbage and any other foods that encourage bacterial fermentation and may trigger intestinal gas.

* Avoid sugar, cakes, sweets and chocolate.

- Try to avoid caffeine-containing drinks such as tea, coffee and soft drinks. Some people are also sensitive to resins in coffee beans, and you may find that drinking decaffeinated coffee can still upset you.
- Try to avoid alcohol as it has a direct irritant effect on the gut.
- Avoid artificial sweeteners such as sorbitol, which are not easily digested and can make symptoms of I.B.S. worse.

Dietary changes to help diarrhoea
- Avoid eating too much raw or dried fruit.
- Avoid spicy foods.
- Cut back on caffeine.
- Avoid artificial sweeteners (especially sorbitol and mannitol).
- Drink plenty of fluids (especially water) to prevent dehydration.
- Eating a live bio yoghurt or a fermented milk drink such as Yakult containing *Lactobacillus acidophilus* can help to replenish the normal bacterial flora of the bowel.
- Eating bananas seems to help.

Dietary changes to help constipation
- In general, aim to eat more fresh fruit, vegetables, salad and pulses.
- Fibre-rich pulses include peas, beans, lentils and chickpeas (garbanzos).
- Eat more fibre-rich dried fruits – especially figs – and seeds, especially sunflower, pumpkin, fenugreek, fennel and linseed. Buy in small quantities with a reasonable sell-by date. Add to salads and yoghurt for an extra crunch.
- Eat more wholegrain cereals: oats, brown rice, wholewheat pasta, wholegrain bread, whole rye, buckwheat, millet, bulgur wheat and couscous.
- Aim to drink one glass (350 ml/12 fl oz) of water before each meal, plus another two or three between meals to bulk up your fibre-rich diet.
- Consider taking a vitamin and mineral supplement containing calcium, magnesium, vitamin C and the B complex.

✤ Natural laxatives include figs, prunes, pears, rhubarb, molasses and linseed.

Kitchen herbs

Many edible natural herbs and spices commonly found in the kitchen can calm the gut, relieve painful spasms and help to prevent wind distension and bloating. Use them as a garnish on food or as soothing herbal teas. Plain infusions of chamomile or peppermint are available in teabags, as are delicious combinations such as chamomile and spearmint or fennel and lemon balm. Useful herbs and spices include the following:

✤ Angelica
✤ Aniseed
✤ Black pepper
✤ Caraway
✤ Chamomile
✤ Clove
✤ Dill
✤ Fennel
✤ Ginger
✤ Lemon balm
✤ Marjoram
✤ Parsley
✤ Peppermint
✤ Rosemary
✤ Spearmint

Dieticians, nutritionists and nutritional therapists

If you experience persistent problems due to I.B.S., you may benefit from dietary advice. If you live in the UK, your GP should be happy to refer you to a dietician. You can also arrange a consultation yourself with any dieticians who see patients privately. State registered dieticians give dietary advice for specific health problems such as I.B.S.

Nutritionists tend to be involved in public health and the scientific study of nutrition, so not all offer individual consultations. You can also seek advice about nutritional supplements from a nutritional therapist. Those with recognized experience, and who have professional indemnity insurance, are registered in the UK with the British Association of Nutritional Therapists. For more information, *see Useful Addresses, page 230.*

CHAPTER 6

I.B.S. and food intolerance

People with I.B.S. whose symptoms are linked to particular foods often feel that a food intolerance, allergy or sensitivity is involved. This is a controversial area, partly because of the way food reactions are classified by doctors. A true food allergy is considered to be either a severe, anaphylactic reaction or a food hypersensitivity. A severe reaction, triggered by specific foods such as peanuts, produces life-threatening symptoms, such as falling blood pressure, difficulty breathing or tissue swelling. In cases of food hypersensitivity, there are symptoms such as a widespread, itchy rash (urticaria), eczema, asthma, vomiting, abdominal pains or diarrhoea when eating specific foods such as strawberries, eggs or shellfish. These two reactions are relatively rare.

Doctors also accept that some people have a food sensitivity in which chemicals found in chocolate, cheese or red wine, for example, can trigger migraine, and that some people have lactose intolerance (due the inability to digest lactose sugar in milk, causing bloating, abdominal pain and diarrhoea) or gluten intolerance (causing bloating, abdominal pain, bulky stools, malabsorption – poor absorption of nutrients in the gut – and weight loss in coeliac disease).

What orthodox medicine finds hard to accept, however, is that other foodstuffs, such as lettuce, corn, yeast, meat, oranges, dairy products or even artificial sweeteners, might cause symptoms of food intolerance in some people, even though this phenomenon appears to be very common. This is because no obvious signs of allergy are found, and because tests performed to help detect food intolerances are not yet accepted as being accurate or reproducible. Even so, as many as one in three people recognize that they cannot eat certain foods without developing problems such as rhinitis (inflammation of the mucous membrane that lines the nose), eczema, headache or digestive symptoms.

Food intolerance testing is now available from a number of pharmacies and health-food shops in the UK. You can order a test kit through Lloyds pharmacies, for example. This will enable you to obtain a pin-prick sample of blood which is then sent to York Nutritional Laboratory. The sample can be screened for reactions to either 40 or 93 different foods.

The British Allergy Foundation recently commissioned an independent, blinded audit of an immune (ELISA) test developed by York Nutritional Laboratories. The results showed that around 52 per cent of those tested who rigorously altered their diet and avoided the foods they were found to react against, experienced a significant reduction in long-term symptoms. A copy of the report is available at www.allergy-testing.com/research.html. According to the Chief Executive of the BAF, 'A tremendous number of people are helped by this test, and a year later, people are still feeling better, having eliminated indicated foods from their diet. A placebo effect would not last this long.' These sensitivities are ill-understood. Further research is undoubtedly needed and clinical trials are underway.

Food intolerance

Food intolerance is defined as a reproducible adverse reaction to a specific food or ingredient, which occurs even when the food is eaten in a disguised form. Many researchers are starting to realize that unrecognized forms of food intolerance are linked with several common, long-term (chronic) problems such as:

- I.B.S.
- Inflammatory bowel diseases
- Premenstrual syndrome
- Chronic fatigue syndrome
- Asthma
- Eczema
- Arthritis

This type of food intolerance has been referred to as 'immuno-antagonism' by some researchers. When food is eaten, it is broken down in the intestines into small building blocks (proteins to amino acids, fats to fatty acids and carbohydrates to simple sugars) before being absorbed. In some cases, however, it is thought that certain foods, to which your immune system is sensitive, make your intestinal wall porous. This is because reactive cells found in the gut lining (mast cells) burst open to attack the food with a cocktail of toxic chemicals. This causes microscopic inflammation in the wall of the gut so that cells swell and move apart, including those in small blood vessels (capillaries), letting incompletely digested food particles (such as chains of amino acids rather than single ones) enter your bloodstream. This theory is supported by research in which proteins from egg yolk and cow's milk have been found in human breast milk. The only logical way in which they could have got there was through the bloodstream. Another possible cause of a leaky gut is an overgrowth of Candida yeast cells, which damage the bowel lining as they grow through layers of cells.

Once in your circulation, food particles to which you are sensitive are quickly attacked by the immune system, coated by immune proteins (complement) and destroyed by white blood cells called neutrophils. If you eat too many of the foods to which you are sensitive, however, it is thought that your immune system becomes swamped. You run out of complement proteins, leaving incompletely-coated food particles free to roam around your body. This challenge to the immune system has been linked with feelings of being tired all the time. The food particles are eventually filtered out in the kidneys and destroyed, but may set up mild inflammation in parts of the body linked with the chronic illnesses mentioned above. At present, this is just a theory and there is no firm evidence to confirm it, although much research continues in the area.

In I.B.S., researchers have suggested that an increased leakiness of the bowel may interfere with its function. There may also be an increase in the level of some hormone-like inflammatory agents (prostaglandins type PGE2) in the rectum, which contribute to the problem. Evening primrose oil may help to balance this out by acting as a building block for making another type of prostaglandin known as the PGE1 series. In some cases, the walls of the colon may become mildly inflamed, swollen and droop a little so that they touch and irritate sensitive muscles near the anus. These muscles interpret the stimulus as a bowel motion ready to be evacuated, and repetitive straining (tenesmus) can occur as the bowel tries to evacuate its floppy walls. This spasm sets up a signal loop that stimulates other parts of the intestines to go into spasm and a vicious circle is set up, leading to spasmodic pain, diarrhoea and intermittent constipation.

Although this all remains theory at present, there is no doubt that many sufferers have symptoms that come on only when certain foods have been eaten. Researchers have found that the people most likely to have a food sensitivity, and whose symptoms will respond to avoiding certain foods, are those with diarrhoea.

Probiotic supplements (*see Chapter 17*), which supply beneficial digestive bacteria, are often helpful in reducing symptoms thought to be due to food sensitivity.

Elimination diet

The diagnosis of food intolerance and allergy can only be made with any degree of reliability when symptoms disappear during an elimination diet and reappear when the suspected food is reintroduced, even in a hidden form. This is best done under proper dietary or medical supervision. There are several degrees of an exclusion diet ranging from:

* Simple exclusion, with the elimination of a single food
* Multiple exclusion – elimination of several foods that have been linked with a particular problem
* Restriction diet – eating very few foods such as nothing but a single meat (e.g. lamb), a single source of carbohydrate (e.g. rice), a single fruit (e.g. pears) and drinking spring, mineral or distilled water

After following the elimination diet until symptoms have disappeared (commonly 10–21 days), the eliminated foods are reintroduced one by one, usually at three-day intervals, to see which triggers a recurrence. You will need to keep a careful food and symptom diary during this time, to help recognize which particular foods, if any, are triggering your symptoms.

Once suspected of causing symptoms, a food should ideally be given in a double-blind, placebo-controlled challenge, meaning that neither the doctor/nurse nor sufferer knows when the suspected food is being given. However, this type of test is very rarely carried out. Food can be disguised or given in liquid form – if necessary through a stomach tube in hospital, for example – when it is felt important to diagnose a food intolerance accurately. You will also be given foods with which you have not previously had a problem to act as a control. If symptoms repeatedly occur only with the disguised suspect food, but not with the control substances, this confirms that the reaction is consistent and a food sensitivity is present. Following an elimination diet, however, is time consuming, can be boring, and requires a great deal of motivation.

BENEFITS OF AN ELIMINATION DIET

A study that looked at the benefits of following an elimination diet found that just under half of I.B.S. sufferers (48 per cent) gained some significant benefit. On average, they were found to be intolerant of between two and five different foods which, when avoided, helped to provide some relief from their symptoms. This would imply that an elimination diet gives you a one in two chance of identifying a problem food and improving symptoms, although they are unlikely to go away altogether.

---

* Avoiding milk-derived foods helps 50 per cent of I.B.S. sufferers
* Cutting out wheat helps 25 per cent
* Cutting out citrus fruits helps 15 per cent
* Avoiding coffee helps 10 per cent

It may be worth cutting out some foods, such as gluten, corn, wheat, coffee, tea, citrus fruits, milk products, for a while and then reintroducing them one at a time to see what happens. Keep a careful food and symptom diary, recording:

- Everything you eat and drink and at what time
- Any symptoms you develop
- At what time symptoms start and how long they last
- Daily activities, stress levels etc.

It may take a few days for a change in diet to affect your symptoms. If you feel there is a definite link with a particular food, keep reintroducing it after avoiding it for several days to confirm that the effect is consistent. If you are fairly confident there is a problem, discuss this with your doctor to ensure that avoiding this food is not going to cause a dietary deficiency. You may also benefit from a referral to a dietician. It is important not to follow an elimination diet for longer than a week or two without professional dietary advice.

If your symptoms are not significantly improved by following a restricted diet, it is important to return to eating a normal diet, and to eating as wide a range of foods as possible, to guard against any nutrient deficiencies. If, however, you are able to identify a small number of foods that undoubtedly provoke your symptoms, these can usually be avoided without affecting your overall nutrition.

ADDENBROOKE'S EXCLUSION DIET

Doctors at Addenbrooke's Hospital, Cambridge, where I trained in medicine, have developed their own exclusion diet for people with I.B.S. On this diet, you are allowed to eat:

- Meat
- Fish
- All fruit except citrus fruits
- Soya products
- All vegetables except potatoes, sweetcorn and onions

You are not allowed to eat or drink:

* Any cereals, except rice
* Any dairy products
* Eggs
* Yeast
* Caffeine
* Nuts
* Alcohol
* Citrus fruits, potatoes, sweetcorn or onions

After following the exclusion diet for a couple of weeks, you can – if you wish – try introducing certain favourite foods (one every three or four days) to see if any are well tolerated without worsening your symptoms. If so, you can continue to keep this food in your diet. If symptoms rapidly worsen, however, that food should be avoided until you feel able to try it again. If symptoms persistently worsen when eating that particular food, and improve when avoiding it, the obvious conclusion is that you are intolerant of it and should consider avoiding it in the long term.

Foods you might want to reintroduce, one at a time, include potatoes, milk, yoghurt, white wine, tea, coffee, cheese, citrus fruits, butter, onions, eggs, chocolate, sweetcorn, wheat, nuts.

The Hay diet

Food combining – also known as the Hay diet – has helped many people with I.B.S. overcome their symptoms. The eating regime is scorned by many food scientists, as there is no obvious theory as to why it works. It is essentially a healthy, wholefood way of eating that increases your fibre intake by concentrating on vegetables, fruit and salads. As it has helped so many people with I.B.S., it may be worth trying if your own symptoms are proving troublesome.

The Hay diet has five basic rules:

1 Fruit, vegetables and salads should make up most of your energy intake
2 Eat only small amounts of carbohydrates
3 When eating carbohydrates, only eat complex, unrefined carbohydrates, such as whole grains – eliminate all refined, processed foods, additives and preservatives
4 Don't eat carbohydrate foods (starches and sugars) at the same mealtime as proteins or fruit acids
5 Allow at least four hours between eating meals of different types

Books explaining the diet in depth and giving sample menu plans are widely available.

CHAPTER 7

I.B.S. and dietary fibre

What is fibre?

Fibre – or roughage – is the term used to describe the indigestible parts of plant foods. It is an essential part of your diet. While fibre provides little in the way of nutritional value, it aids the digestion and absorption of other foods. Fibre provides important bulk for the bowel to grip onto and push downwards. It therefore encourages peristalsis (the muscular, wave-like motion which transports digested food through the intestines) and helps to regulate bowel voiding.

Fibre is an essential component of all plant cell structures. We lack the enzymes necessary to break down fibre in the intestines but gut bacteria can ferment fibre in the bowel. This process does release a lot of gas, however, which will make symptoms of I.B.S. worse for some people.

Experiments show that for every 1 gram of fibre you eat, your bowel motions increase by around 5 grams. This is because dietary fibre provides nutrients for bacterial growth, and much of the increased bowel motion bulk is due to increased bacterial multiplication in the gut. Fibre also absorbs water and toxins from the gut, which increases stool bulk and weight.

SOLUBLE AND INSOLUBLE FIBRE

There are two main types of dietary fibre: soluble and insoluble.

Soluble fibre is important in the stomach and upper intestines, where it slows down the processes of digestion and absorption. This ensures that blood sugar and fat levels rise only slowly, so the body can handle nutrient fluctuations more easily.

Insoluble fibre is most important in the large bowel. It bulks up the faeces, absorbs water and hastens stool excretion. In general, soluble fibre is totally broken down in the large bowel, while insoluble fibre is passed out in the motions.

All plant foods contain both soluble and insoluble fibre, though some sources are richer in one type than another. The table below gives some common examples of foods rich in dietary fibre.

Sources of soluble and insoluble fibre

Classification	Plant source	A few examples
SOLUBLE	Oats	Porridge, muesli
	Barley	Pearl barley
	Rye	Rye bread, crispbread
	Fruit	Figs, apricots, tomatoes, apples
	Vegetables	Carrots, potatoes, courgettes (zucchini)
	Pulses	Cannellini beans, kidney beans
INSOLUBLE	Wheat	Wholemeal bread, cereals
	Maize	Sweetcorn, corn bread
	Rice	Brown rice
	Pasta	Wholemeal pasta, spinach pasta
	Fruit	Rhubarb, blackberries, strawberries
	Vegetables	Cabbage, spinach, lettuce
	Pulses	Peas, lentils, chickpeas (garbanzos)

Dietary fibre and I.B.S.

Some people with I.B.S., especially those with constipation, find that eating a high-fibre diet improves their symptoms. Sometimes it takes a few weeks for benefits to be felt, however, and symptoms may worsen before they improve.

If you don't eat enough fibre, the reabsorption of nutrients and fluid from bowel motions results in very little bulk reaching the lower colon for propulsion towards the rectum. Instead of the small muscular contractions needed to move bulky stools downwards (peristalsis), the colon walls have to squeeze tightly to propel the smaller pellets on their way. This is thought to lead to prolonged muscle spasms and the pain associated with some cases of I.B.S. – especially the type known as spastic colon syndrome. When the bowel is in spasm, any additional emotional or physical stress will prolong the symptoms and aggravate the pain, as receptors in the bowel wall are sensitive to stress hormones, which may also be released as a result of pain.

A low-fibre diet can lead to constipation. Small, hard, pellet-like stools form when bowel contents stay in contact with the intestinal walls for longer than usual so that more fluid is reabsorbed. The lack of bulk can also produce diarrhoea if there is not enough fibre to absorb excess fluid.

There is no consistent link, however, between a sufferer's symptoms of I.B.S. and fibre intake. It is unlikely that a single dietary factor, such as lack of fibre, is the sole cause. Increasing fibre intake to between 15 and 30 grams (½ to 1 ounce) per day will usually help to relieve constipation (especially in patients with spastic colon syndrome).

Overall, following a high-fibre diet helps around one-third of people with I.B.S. In up to a quarter of sufferers, however, changing to a high-fibre diet initially makes the bloating and distension of I.B.S. worse. This effect disappears after two or three weeks, so it's worth trying to persevere and to build up your fibre intake slowly so your bowel has time to get used to it. When increasing fibre intake, add in a probiotic supplement to ensure a healthy balance of bacteria to ferment fibre in the lower bowel.

If fibre does help you, it is important to eat as many different sources of fibre as possible. New research suggests that bowel bacteria quickly adapt to the types of roughage in your diet. If you mainly eat fibre of one type (such as a bran supplement), your colonic bacteria will respond within a week or two by increasing their output of enzymes needed to ferment this. The fibre reaching your colon will then be broken down more quickly, so that even if a high-fibre diet has initially helped your symptoms, you will lose much of the benefit gained and your symptoms may return.

It is very important to drink plenty of water when eating a high-fibre diet, as this helps the fibre swell in the intestines so it can work properly. Fibre in the bowel absorbs large quantities of water. If fluid intake is inadequate, the fibre will dry out and irritate the bowel wall, which may cause spasm and pain.

Some people find that fibre consistently makes their symptoms worse. This is sometimes due to a condition known as 'complex carbohydrate intolerance' (CCI), in which a high-fibre diet produces problematic symptoms resulting from intestinal wind. This is thought to occur when the small intestine does not produce all the enzymes needed to completely digest carbohydrate-rich foods. In such cases, a low-fibre diet may be the answer. The best option is to increase your fibre intake slowly over a week or so, and to maintain the higher intake for a further three or four weeks. If, after a month, your symptoms are not improved, cut back and try a low-fibre diet for a similar length of time to assess which suits you best.

ALTERNATIVES TO BRAN
In one study of 100 patients:

- 55 per cent said bran made their symptoms worse
- 10 per cent said bran helped

Of those whose symptoms worsened, 67 per cent rated their deterioration as substantial, while 33 per cent said it was moderate. If you cannot tolerate bran – as at least half of I.B.S. sufferers can't – taking supplements containing other, more gentle forms of fibre, such as psyllium or flaxseed, is often effective.

Chapter 8

I.B.S. and wheat

Many people with I.B.S. find their symptoms become worse when eating wheat or wheat bran products. When wheat is eliminated from their diet, symptoms improve. This may, however, be due to altering the total amount of bran fibre in their diet rather than to a wheat sensitivity itself.

Wheat also contains gluten, so if a wheat-free diet improves your symptoms, you should also consider avoiding other gluten-containing foods to see if this improves symptoms even more. If your symptoms improve dramatically, it is possible that you have an undiagnosed gluten intolerance (known as coeliac disease), rather than I.B.S., and your doctor can assess whether or not you need further investigations to confirm this.

Not everyone with I.B.S. who does not tolerate wheat well will have coeliac disease. Some people seem to be unusually sensitive to other components of wheat, such as wheat bran. It is therefore worth experimenting to see whether avoiding wheat products is beneficial for you.

Gluten intolerance

Gluten is a protein found in several cereals, including wheat, rye, barley and possibly some types of oats. Coeliac disease (gluten sensitive enteropathy), which can come on at any age, is relatively common, affecting around one person in 2000 (in Ireland it is more prevalent, and affects one person in 300). Coeliac disease affects more females than males and often runs in families. Classically, sufferers are said to be fair-haired and blue-eyed, although this is not always the case. If symptoms develop in childhood, the sufferer is often shorter than expected due to poor absorption of nutrients from the gut. In adults, gluten sensitivity most often develops in the thirties and forties.

Symptoms of coeliac disease vary. Some sufferers develop few problems and are unaware of their condition. Others experience a variety of symptoms that can creep up over months or years, such as:

* Tiredness
* Generalized feelings of being unwell
* Breathlessness
* Abdominal pain
* Bloating and wind
* Diarrhoea
* Vomiting
* Passing pale, bulky, offensive, fatty stools that float (steatorrhoea)
* Weight loss
* Mouth ulcers and sores at the corner of the mouth
* Skin changes including pigmentation, scaliness, easy bruising and a rash known as *Dermatitis herpetiformis,* although those with skin symptoms tend not to develop the abdominal symptoms of coeliac disease

The symptoms of coeliac disease are due to abnormal changes in a part of the small intestine known as the jejunum.

THE JEJUNUM

The first part of the small intestine forms a tube known as the jejunum. The inner lining of the jejunum is covered in tiny, finger-like projections around a millimetre long, known as villi. These increase the surface area of the intestinal wall to speed up absorption of the products of digestion, including vitamins, and fluid. After digestion, nutrients pass into the villi where they enter tiny blood capillaries for transportation to the liver or into small lymph vessels, called lacteals, for distribution into the lymph system. The small intestines process around 9 litres (16 pints) of fluid per day – 2 litres

(3½ pints) from your diet and 7 litres (12 pints) secreted in the form of digestive juices. Only 1–2 litres of fluid are passed through into the large bowel, however. The rest is absorbed in the small intestines.

In coeliac disease, the villi disappear from the lining of the jejunum, which becomes abnormally smooth. As a result, absorption of fluids and nutrients is reduced so that half of all people with the condition have mild anaemia (due to iron and/or folic acid deficiency). These changes in the jejunal lining are brought on by exposure to dietary gluten, and are due to a hypersensitivity to gliadin, a small protein (polypeptide) found in gluten. This may be a direct toxic effect or be triggered by an over-zealous immune system – possibly brought on in susceptible people by exposure to a particular virus (Adenovirus 12). When following a gluten-free diet, the villi redevelop and symptoms disappear, but will quickly return whenever gluten-containing foods are eaten. Coeliac disease is therefore a condition totally dependent on dietary intake.

DIAGNOSIS OF COELIAC DISEASE

If coeliac disease is suspected, it is possible to perform a special blood allergy test to detect antibodies against gliadin, the small protein (polypeptide) found in gluten, to which sufferers are sensitive. A sample of blood fluid (serum) is split, diluted and incubated with special beads that are pre-coated with gliadin. If antibodies are present in the person's blood, they will bind to the gliadin on the beads. In the next step, the beads are washed and then exposed to fluorescent antibodies that will, in turn, react with any antibody previously bound to the beads (i.e. they are anti-human antibody antibodies!). If antibody is present in the patient's blood, the beads will then fluoresce bright green when looked at under the microscope to give a positive test. This test is not yet widely available and may give false positives in some patients with other illnesses involving the gut, such as cystic fibrosis or Crohn's disease.

The diagnosis of coeliac disease can also be confirmed by taking a biopsy of the small intestine. This involves swallowing a small, cylindrical metal device attached to 2 metres (6½ feet) of polyethylene tubing. Its position is monitored by x-ray or positioned using an endoscopic viewing instrument. When the capsule is in the jejunum, a spring-loaded knife-blade within the capsule snips off a tiny piece of the bowel lining. The capsule is then gently pulled back up through the gut to retrieve the sample. If coeliac disease is present, the biopsy obtained will show abnormal smoothness of the jejunal lining, instead of the normal tiny projections (villi). Signs of inflammation will also be present. The biopsy is usually repeated up to three times – once when following a gluten-containing diet, secondly when following a gluten-free diet and thirdly when eating gluten again to confirm the diagnosis.

Although the majority of people with symptoms of I.B.S. do not have coeliac disease, the condition can be misdiagnosed as I.B.S. If you think there is a possibility that you have gluten sensitivity, try following a gluten-free diet for a few weeks to see if your symptoms improve. If they do, discuss the possibility with your doctor. If coeliac disease is confirmed, you will need to follow a gluten-free diet for life.

Vitamins and minerals
If you have coeliac disease and have had delayed diagnosis, or do not follow a strict gluten-free diet, you will have a reduced absorption of many vitamins and minerals. This can lead to anaemia due to lack of iron and/or folic acid. A good idea as a nutritional safety net is a complete vitamin and mineral supplement providing at least 100 per cent of the recommended daily amount (RDA) of as many micronutrients as possible.

Gluten-free diet
Gluten-free versions of cereal-containing foods such as bread and cakes are widely available. In the UK, you can also obtain gluten-free products on prescription from your doctor. Check food labels carefully for hidden gluten, as wheat is often present in products such as soups, stock cubes and dessert mixes.

On a gluten-free diet you can eat:

* Fruit, salads and vegetables, including potatoes
* Soya bran, rice bran
* Rice, tapioca, sago, arrowroot, buckwheat, millet, maize, corn
* Fresh or frozen (unprocessed) meat, poultry, offal
* Plain (uncoated) fish (fresh or frozen)
* Eggs, plain cheese
* Milk, cream, butter, margarine and oils
* Yoghurts and fromage frais (except those containing muesli or cereals)
* Nuts and seeds
* Gluten-free flour, soya flour, potato flour, pea flour, rice flour
* Bread, crispbread and pasta products that are labelled as gluten-free
* Gluten-free biscuits, cakes
* Gluten-free breakfast cereals
* Sugar, jam, marmalade, honey, jelly
* Herbs, spices, mustard, vinegar, salt, pepper
* Tea, coffee, fruit juice
* Wine, beer, spirits

On a gluten-free diet you must avoid:

* Wheat bran
* Breakfast cereals containing wheat or oats
* Barley, oatmeal, semolina
* Ordinary (gluten-containing) bread, crispbread, pasta
* Ordinary flour, rye flour, barley flour, pastry made from these
* Ordinary biscuits and cakes
* Pastry, pies etc.
* Meat pies, beefburgers, sausages, tinned meats
* Fish in breadcrumbs, batter, fishcakes, fish fingers etc.
* Scotch eggs
* Potato croquettes
* Tinned and refined foods using wheat flour as a thickener
* Most stock cubes, gravy mixes etc.
* Barley water and some night-time drinks

Avoid any food labelled as containing:

* Malt
* Rye
* Rusk
* Barley
* Oats
* Food starch
* Flour starch
* Edible starch
* Modified starch
* Wheat starch
* Wheat flour
* Cereal filler
* Cereal binder
* Cereal protein
* Vegetable protein

You should also check that all medicines are gluten-free.

CHAPTER 9

I.B.S. and yeasts

Symptoms of I.B.S. have been linked with the yeast-like fungus, *Candida albicans*. Candida usually lives quite happily in and on the body of a large proportion of the population without causing harm. When in its harmless form, it is present as simple yeast cells that grow and reproduce by putting out small buds that break off to form new daughter cells. Studies have shown that Candida can be found in:

* The mouth of up to 1 in 2 healthy people
* The oesophagus (gullet) of 1 in 10 healthy volunteers
* The duodenal secretions of 1 in 25 healthy people
* The jejunum of 1 in 2 apparently normal and healthy adults
* The colon and faeces of 8 out of 10 people
* The rectum of 1 in 3 people

It is likely that everyone has Candida growing in their gut at some time during each year – if not permanently. It is usually kept under control and stopped from over-growing by a variety of factors including:

* Competition for nutrients by bowel bacteria
* Secretion of natural anti-fungal agents by bowel bacteria
* Bowel enzymes and juices
* The action of antibodies secreted onto the inner gut lining
* Immune cells that patrol the bowel wall

Acting together, these different factors usually damp down Candida growth so that it lives quite happily inside you – and may even do some good. Vitamins made by yeast cells – especially the B group and biotin – seep into your intestinal juices and are readily absorbed, for example. If environmental conditions change, however, Candida can switch from its harmless (commensal) form to put out germ tubes (hyphae) that can invade local tissues. This usually occurs only if your natural immunity is weakened through:

* Taking broad-spectrum antibiotics
* Poor nutrition
* Serious illness, such as cancer, AIDS
* Taking drugs that lower immunity, such as chemotherapy, systemic corticosteroids, drugs used in organ transplantation

Even so, some apparently well people have been found to have symptoms linked with Candida overgrowth in the small intestine, and the reason why they overgrow is unknown.

Symptoms of Candida overgrowth

If Candida overgrows and invades the wall of the gut, it can cause symptoms such as:

* Sensitivity to certain foods
* Flatulence
* Bloating
* Nausea
* Vomiting bile-stained fluids
* Abdominal pain
* Diarrhoea – usually watery, explosive, without blood or mucus, and comes and goes over several weeks
* Ulceration of the intestinal wall leading to bleeding (blood lost from this part of the bowel will usually be dark red/brown/black) by the time it reaches the anus

One study reported six cases of small bowel candidiasis in adults, five of whom had no obvious underlying illness or immune problem, and only two of whom had recently taken antibiotics. The main symptom was diarrhoea that lasted from four days to three months. As soon as a course of anti-fungal treatment (nystatin) was started, symptoms disappeared within three to four days.

In another study, 50 adults with recurrent diarrhoea and a variety of gastro-intestinal symptoms were found to have a heavy growth of *Candida albicans* in their stool, which was thought to be the cause of their problem.

Many people with I.B.S. develop symptoms for the first time after an attack of gastroenteritis (bowel infection), which disrupts bowel flora and may make it easier for Candida to overgrow. During 1994, 38 victims of an outbreak of salmonella food poisoning were studied by researchers and over the next year, almost a third went on to develop recurrent bowel symptoms consistent with I.B.S.

Another study looked at 75 patients who developed gastroenteritis from various organisms that was bad enough for them to be admitted to hospital. Of these, 22 had symptoms three months later that were consistent with I.B.S. Nine out of ten of these were still suffering after six months, and three-quarters still had I.B.S. problems one year later (*see page 10*).

Researchers are unclear why bacterial bowel infections are linked with I.B.S., but a sensitivity to Candida products, or to a resultant yeast overgrowth which somehow interferes with normal bowel function, have been suggested.

Candida and food sensitivity

While an overgrowth of Candida in the small intestine produces obvious inflammation that can be diagnosed and treated, the presence of non-invasive (harmless) Candida in the gut is now thought to be linked with an allergic hypersensitivity reaction that can trigger symptoms of I.B.S. – especially diarrhoea – in certain people. This may occur after taking antibiotics. Where skin tests have linked recurrent diarrhoea with hypersensitivity to yeast cells, and where Candida have been cultured from stool samples, bowel symptoms have been shown to get worse in patients given Candida extracts to eat. Treatment to wipe out bowel Candida infection, plus a yeast-free diet, can help.

In many cases, however, anti-Candida treatment does not improve symptoms. Rather than dismissing Candida as a cause, researchers should instead look for another explanation in which Candida may play a role. It may be that an overgrowth of Candida has damaged the bowel wall enough to make it leaky, so that other chemicals – including partially digested food particles – that do not usually reach the bloodstream are absorbed. This may set up an immune response known as immuno-antagonism (*see page 61*), in which case the presence of Candida has acted as a trigger for I.B.S., but has not caused it directly. Once the damage is done and the bowel and immune system are sensitized to these food particles, treatment to eradicate the yeast overgrowth would not be expected to help.

Type of food	Number of samples tested	Number positive for live Candida yeasts	%
Drinks	16	4	25
Breads	8	0	0
Cereals	17	2	12
Condiments	23	0	0
Desserts	39	1	3
Fish	4	0	0
Fruits	6	0	0
Juices	61	38	62
Meats (cooked)	20	0	0
Milk and products	27	1	4
Salads	8	3	38
Sauces	10	0	0
Snacks	25	3	12
Soups	16	0	0
Vegetables	44	2	5
Ready-cooked meals	21	0	0

Anti-Candida diet

While this area remains controversial, some researchers have linked I.B.S. symptoms with a sensitivity to Candida yeasts in the gut. Candida yeasts mostly enter your gut through the mouth, especially in the food you eat. Following an anti-Candida diet is designed to reduce the chance of ingesting yeast cells, and to limit the growth of those already present in your bowel. This is not always easy, however, as live Candida yeasts are frequently present in food and drinks. In one study that analysed a range of common foods, live Candida cells were recovered from a number of items.

With the juices, all vegetable and fruit types were affected, including apple, pineapple, orange, tomato, grape, apricot and lemonade. The yeast contamination seemed to be related to the type of packaging and processing used during preparation rather than the type of fruit involved. All juices sealed with foil wraps were contaminated, while those in cans or bottles were yeast-free (*see table page 80*).

There is no doubt that many people with I.B.S. notice a significant improvement in their symptoms if they follow a low-yeast, anti-Candida diet. This involves avoiding products containing brewers' or bakers' yeast, and products that promote their growth, such as refined carbohydrates and sugar:

* Avoid refined carbohydrates (e.g. white flour) and products made from them. You should also generally reduce your intake of carbohydrates. This goes against most healthy-eating guidance (which encourages you to eat more unrefined, complex carbohydrates), so if you have not noticed a significant benefit from the diet after a few weeks, it is important to return to a normal pattern of healthy eating.
* Avoid white or brown sugar and food and drinks containing them (e.g. honey, jam, desserts, treacle, cakes, biscuits, sauces, ice-cream, soft drinks, dried fruits, chocolates etc).
* Avoid products containing yeast, such as yeast extracts, cheese, bread made with yeast, alcoholic drinks, vinegar and pickled foods, grapes and grape juice, unpeeled fruits, dried fruits, frozen or concentrated fruit juices, old potentially-mouldy foods, mushrooms, B-vitamin supplements that are not labelled 'yeast-free'.

✿ Eat lots of foods that contain natural anti-fungal agents, such as garlic, herbs and spices, fresh green leafy vegetables.

If you are not overweight and find you start losing more than one or two pounds on the above regime, it is important to seek nutritional advice from a dietician. This can be arranged through your own doctor.

How to boost your immune system
To give your immune system a general boost without sticking to an anti-Candida regime:

✿ Follow a wholefood diet containing plenty of peeled fresh fruit, vegetables and wholegrains, with as few processed foods and additives as possible.
✿ Cut back on your intake of omega-6 polyunsaturated vegetable fats (found in margarine, cakes, biscuits etc.) and eat more omega-3 essential fatty acids (such as those found in oily fish).
✿ Take a good vitamin and mineral supplement providing as many vitamins and minerals as possible at around 100 per cent of the recommended daily amount (RDA).
✿ Consider taking higher doses of the antioxidant vitamins C and E.
✿ Consider taking pure evening primrose oil supplements.
✿ If you smoke, do your utmost to stop.
✿ Limit your alcohol intake to no more than one to two units per day.
✿ Eat live (unpasteurized) bio yoghurt containing organisms such as Lactobacilli or Bifidobacteria species to help colonize your bowel with friendly bacteria *(see page 190)*.
✿ Take a supplement providing prebiotics, such as fructo-oligosaccharides (FOS) *(see page 190)*.
✿ Take regular exercise.
✿ Obtain adequate rest and sleep.

CHAPTER 10

I.B.S. and dairy products

Milk contains special proteins, such as casein, and a sugar, lactose, that can trigger food intolerance in some people. Milk protein allergy is mainly found in children and is linked to diarrhoea and eczema. Most grow out of it, and it is unusual to find milk protein sensitivity in adults, even in those suffering from I.B.S.

Lactose intolerance, however, is relatively common and is due to a metabolic deficiency of an enzyme, lactase, needed to digest lactose before it can be absorbed. Lactase enzyme is released from the lining of the small intestine and acts on a molecule of lactose to break it down into two sugars, glucose and galactose, which are immediately absorbed into the bloodstream. Lactase deficiency leads to similar symptoms as those seen in I.B.S., which can include:

* Bloating and wind
* Audible bowel sounds (borborygmi)
* Abdominal pain
* Diarrhoea

Lactase deficiency can be present from birth (primary lactase deficiency) or can result temporarily after a bout of gastroenteritis (secondary lactase deficiency).

Testing for lactose intolerance

Lactase deficiency is sometimes diagnosed by taking a lactose tolerance test. In the classic test, a solution containing a known amount of lactose is taken by mouth. A blood sample is taken at the beginning of the test, then at various intervals to assess blood sugar levels. Symptoms such as bowel distension, pain, flatulence and diarrhoea are also noted throughout the test. If blood sugar levels fail to rise above a certain level, lactose digestion and absorption is abnormal and implies a deficiency of lactase enzyme. Results can be difficult to interpret if sugar diabetes is present, however.

Another test, the ethanol galactose test, involves giving a known dose of alcohol followed by lactose sugar solution. A blood sample is taken at the beginning of the test and again after 40 minutes, and blood galactose levels are measured. A rise in blood galactose of less than 5 mg/100 ml is considered abnormal and implies lactose digestion and absorption is faulty.

A more reliable test is to measure breath hydrogen levels after a known amount of a carbohydrate, such as lactose, is eaten. In normal conditions, the hydrogen content of the breath does not increase as all lactose is absorbed. If there is a deficiency of lactase, the sugar reaches the colon where bowel bacteria ferment it to produce an increase in breath hydrogen content after around 90 minutes of eating.

In a modification of this test, lactose labelled with a safe radioactive carbon atom is given. Air samples are then collected at hourly intervals to see how much radioactive labelled carbon dioxide gas is breathed out. This test is one of the most accurate available, but it is expensive and only usually used by well-funded researchers.

Alternatively, a small bowel (jejunal) biopsy (*see page 73*) can be taken to provide a definitive answer as to whether someone has lactose intolerance. The biopsy tissue is broken up and incubated in a solution containing lactose to accurately measure how much lactase enzyme activity is present.

Lactose-free diet

Treatment of lactose intolerance involves following a lactose elimination diet in which soya or low-lactose milk products are used in place of cow's milk:

Lactose content of different milks	
	Lactose (g) per glass
Sheep's milk	9.9 g (avoid)
Skimmed cow's milk	9.8 g (avoid)
Full fat cow's milk	9.3 g (avoid)
Goat's milk	8.6 g (avoid)
Low-lactose cow's milk	0.5 g
Soya milk	0 g

Yoghurt made from cow's milk has a low lactose content as bacterial fermentation breaks the lactose down.

If avoiding cow's milk products, you will need to ensure you are getting an adequate intake of vitamins A and D and the mineral calcium from alternative sources, including supplements. Good dietary sources of calcium other than dairy milk products include:

* Calcium-enriched soya milk
* Eggs
* Green leafy vegetables, such as broccoli and spinach
* Whitebait, tinned salmon and sardines, which include soft bones
* Nuts, such as almonds, brazils, hazelnuts
* Seeds, such as sesame, tahini
* Pulses, such as chickpeas (garbanzos), beans, lentils, soybeans and products (such as tofu)
* White and brown bread – in the UK, white and brown flours are fortified with calcium by law, but not wholemeal flour which already has a good calcium content
* Dried or fresh figs
* Oranges
* Prawns, cockles, mussels

Recent research suggests that it may not be beneficial to investigate people with I.B.S. for lactose intolerance, even if their symptoms improve on a low-lactose diet. When 122 people with I.B.S. (37 male,

85 female) were given lactose hydrogen breath tests, those with a positive test followed a low-lactose diet for three weeks. Those whose symptoms improved on the diet were then challenged with lactose in varying doses or given a placebo. Those who did not respond to the low-lactose diet were asked to follow an exclusion diet, or a low-fibre diet instead.

Of those who tested positive for lactose intolerance, 27 per cent experienced significantly worse I.B.S. symptoms after the test, presumably as a result of the test. Following a low-lactose diet produced disappointing results in those shown to have lactose intolerance, and milk intolerance was found to cause problems for people in both groups. The researchers therefore felt there was little advantage in trying to separate people with I.B.S. into those who were intolerant of lactose from those who were not. It seems to be just as effective to try different eating approaches (dairy-free, lactose-free, low-fibre or exclusion diet) to find which suits you best without going to the trouble and worry of tests.

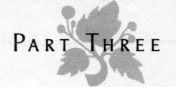

PART THREE

The Recipes

As you will have gathered from the book so far, there is a high chance that what you eat will have an effect on your I.B.S. symptoms. The last thing you want, however, is to become so worried about your diet that you starve yourself for fear of eating something which will disagree with you. Neither do you want to waste time and energy preparing complicated 'special diet' dishes. The recipes that follow are quick and easy to make. They take account of fibre content and avoid accepted triggers and allergens, but can still be enjoyably eaten by anyone, whether or not they have I.B.S.

Fibre

As you will realize by now, some people with I.B.S. do well on a high-fibre diet, but this can spell disaster for others. I have therefore included high-fibre and low-fibre dishes, as well as some in the middle. An indication of the fibre content is included in the introduction to each recipe. When the dish is high in fibre, I have tried to specify the high-fibre ingredient so that you can adapt the recipe if you need to.

Gluten

Since gluten causes problems for a large number of I.B.S. sufferers, I have excluded it from the recipes almost entirely by substituting rice, chickpea, potato, maize and other gluten-free grains or flours. If you do not have a problem with wheat or gluten, you may replace the alternative grains in most recipes with wheat, although it might be a good idea to experiment with some of these alternative flours and grains – all of which actually taste very good – in the interests of achieving as wide a diet as possible. Recipes are flagged up as being gluten- and/or wheat-free.

Lactose

Many I.B.S. sufferers also react badly to lactose, the natural form of sugar found in cow's milk. I have therefore excluded all primary, or unprocessed, dairy products from the recipes. The fermentation needed to create yoghurt or fromage frais breaks down the lactose sugar in milk, making it relatively easy to digest, so I use both products fairly liberally. You might want to experiment with products made from alternatives to cow's milk, such as goat, sheep or buffalo milk, which many people find more digestible. There is now a wide range of non-animal milks, such as soya, oat, rice, peanut and coconut, which work very well in most dishes. Recipes are flagged as being dairy-free (containing no cow's milk) or as having the possibility of being dairy-free. If you do not have a problem with dairy products, you can use cow's milk wherever milk is specified.

Candida

Since Candida may be a factor in many people's I.B.S., I have avoided using yeast in any recipes and, wherever possible, have used puréed fruits as an alternative to refined sugar in the desserts and baking recipes. Puréed fruits have the further advantage of adding fibre to an otherwise low-fibre dish.

Omega-3 fatty acids

Many I.B.S. sufferers have a depressed immune system. As a boost, I have included a number of dishes based on oily fish, such as salmon, mackerel, sardines, tuna and anchovies. These will not only boost your intake of omega-3s, but also your intake of calcium.

Fresh fruit and vegetables

The vast majority of the recipes are either based on, or contain, substantial quantities of fresh fruits and vegetables. Always make sure your fruit and vegetables are as fresh as possible and washed thoroughly. If you can find, and afford, organic produce, so much the better. Although there is as yet little research to suggest that organic food is nutritionally better than non-organic, protecting delicate digestive systems from even the tiniest residues of chemical fertilizers and pesticides seems like a sensible idea.

I hope that you find the recipes quick and easy to prepare, and enjoy them as much as I did when testing them. Happy cooking!

MICHELLE BERRIEDALE-JOHNSON

CHAPTER 11

Soups and starters

Cream of Mushroom Soup
with Anchovies

Cutting animal milks out of your diet need not mean the end of cream soups. Alternatives such as soya, oat or rice milk work very well when cooked, while puréeing can give you a cream soup without any milk at all. The anchovies in this soup should give plenty of flavour, so there's no need to add extra salt. This soup is also suitable for those on low-fibre diets.

N.B. If you prefer your mushroom soup really 'bitty', you do not need to purée it at all.

Ingredients SERVES 4

METRIC (IMPERIAL)	AMERICAN
3 tablespoons olive oil	3 tablespoons
4 tinned anchovies with their oil, chopped small	4
1 large leek, thinly sliced	1 large
450g (1lb) mushrooms of your choice, sliced thinly	1lb
1 tablespoon potato flour or cornflour (cornstarch)	1 tablespoon
400ml (14fl oz) oat or soya milk	1¾ cups
750ml (1¼ pints) gluten- and wheat-free chicken or vegetable stock, homemade if possible	3 cups
juice of 1 lemon	juice of 1
freshly ground black pepper	
2 tablespoons walnut oil	2 tablespoons
1 tablespoon pine nuts	1 tablespoon

Method

1 Gently heat the olive oil in a deep, heavy pan.

2 Add the anchovies, leek and 400g (14oz) of the mushrooms.

3 Cover the pan and sweat gently for 15 minutes or until all the vegetables are soft.

4 Add the potato flour or cornflour (cornstarch), stir around for a couple of minutes, then add the oat or soya milk and the stock. Bring to the boil then reduce heat and simmer for 30–40 minutes.

5 Purée the mixture in a food processor then return to the pan. Season with the lemon juice and freshly ground black pepper.

6 Gently heat the walnut oil in a separate pan and add the pine nuts and the remaining mushrooms. Cook for a few minutes until the mushrooms are just softened and the pine nuts coloured. Add to the soup just before serving.

Tomato and Sweet Potato Soup

Wheat/gluten-free 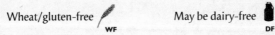 **WF**   May be dairy-free **DF**

This soup is gloriously golden – and has the advantage of being very easy to make and almost fat-free. However, it is also quite high in fibre and provides lots of vitamins C and E. You can serve it as it is or 'dress it up' with seeds or a dollop or yoghurt or fromage frais.

Ingredients

SERVES 4

METRIC (IMPERIAL)	AMERICAN
2 medium leeks, peeled and sliced thickly	2 medium
300g (11oz) sweet potato, peeled and diced	11oz
400g (14oz) tinned tomatoes in their own juice	14oz
600ml (1 pint) water or gluten- and wheat-free vegetable or chicken stock	2½ cups
4 tablespoons fresh/tinned/frozen (defrosted) corn kernels	4 tablespoons
salt, pepper and Tabasco	

Optional extras

1 tablespoon toasted sunflower or sesame seeds *or*	1 tablespoon
4 teaspoons creamy plain yoghurt or fromage frais	4 teaspoons
pinch paprika	pinch

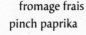

Method

1 Put the leeks in a large pan with the sweet potatoes, tomatoes and water or stock.
2 Bring to the boil and simmer gently until the sweet potato and leeks are quite soft.
3 Purée thoroughly in a food processor or liquidizer.
4 Add the corn kernels and season with salt, pepper and Tabasco to taste. If the soup is too thick, thin it with a little extra water or stock.
5 Serve either as it is or sprinkled with sunflower or sesame seeds – or with a teaspoon of yoghurt or fromage frais in each bowl, sprinkled with a tiny pinch of paprika pepper.

Leek and Lettuce Soup with Butterbeans

Wheat/gluten-free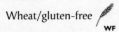
WF

Dairy-free
DF

A versatile and tasty soup, which can be served hot or cold. It is also relatively high in fibre, with around 3g per portion.

Ingredients

SERVES 4

METRIC (IMPERIAL)	AMERICAN
3 tablespoons virgin olive or sunflower oil	3 tablespoons
3 large leeks, trimmed and sliced thinly	3 large
1 medium cos (romaine) lettuce, sliced thickly	1 medium
300g (11oz) tinned butterbeans (reserve liquid)	11oz
750ml (1¼ pints) soya or oat milk	3 cups
sea salt and freshly ground black pepper	
handful chives	handful

Method

1 Put the oil, leeks and lettuce in a deep, heavy pan, cover and sweat for 20–30 minutes, until the leeks are thoroughly cooked.
2 Add the butterbeans, together with the liquid in the tin, and milk, and purée the mixture in a food processor or liquidizer.
3 Season to taste with sea salt and freshly ground black pepper.
4 The soup can be served either hot or cold but sprinkle with finely chopped chives just before serving.

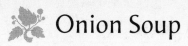

Onion Soup

Wheat/gluten-free 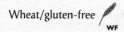 **WF**   May be dairy-free **DF**

Slow-cooked onion soup is one of the most delicious dishes, especially on a cold winter's night. If you are on a low-fibre diet, the long cooking time will make the vegetables more easily digestible.

Ingredients

SERVES 4

METRIC (IMPERIAL)	AMERICAN
2 tablespoons olive oil	2 tablespoons
450g (1lb) sweet Spanish onions, peeled and sliced fairly thickly	1lb
1 tablespoon fresh thyme *or*	1 tablespoon
½ tablespoon dried thyme	½ tablespoon
3 cloves garlic	3 cloves
900ml (1½ pints) chicken stock	3¾ cups
sea salt and black peppercorns	

Optional extras

1 tablespoon pine nuts or sesame seeds, lightly toasted under a grill or on a griddle *or*	1 tablespoon
4 teaspoons fromage frais	4 teaspoons

Method

1 Heat the oil in a heavy-based saucepan. Add the onions, thyme and garlic. Cover and sweat very gently, without burning, for 45 minutes.

2 Add the chicken stock, a pinch of salt and 6–8 black peppercorns, lightly crushed with a rolling pin. Bring to the boil then reduce heat and simmer for a further 30–40 minutes.

3 Adjust the seasoning to taste.

4 Spoon the soup into bowls. Serve as it is or add a sprinkling of pine nuts, sesame seeds or a teaspoon of fromage frais.

Chicken and Courgette (Small Zucchini) Soup

Wheat/gluten-free 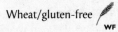 **WF**   May be dairy-free **DF**

This soup is a good, tasty and relatively low-fibre way to use up leftover chicken. The fresh herbs are a colourful and flavoursome addition.

Ingredients   SERVES 4

METRIC (IMPERIAL)	AMERICAN
2 tablespoons olive oil	2 tablespoons
2 medium onions, peeled and chopped roughly	2 medium
2 medium courgettes (small zucchini), sliced	2 medium
1 teaspoon dried thyme	1 teaspoon
150g (5oz) cooked chicken, chopped	5oz
1 litre (1¾ pints) gluten- and wheat-free chicken or vegetable stock	4¼ cups
salt and pepper	
1 tablespoon fresh coriander or parsley, chopped	1 tablespoon
4 teaspoons yoghurt (optional)	4 teaspoons

Method

1 Heat the oil in a deep pan and cook the onions and courgettes (small zucchini) with the thyme until soft.
2 Add the chicken and stock and bring to the boil. Reduce the heat and simmer for 15–20 minutes.
3 Purée in a food processor and adjust the seasoning to taste.
4 To serve, reheat thoroughly until piping hot and sprinkle with the chopped coriander or parsley. If you wish to use the yoghurt, swirl a spoonful into each bowl before sprinkling with the chopped herbs.

Aubergine (Eggplant) and Smoked Fish Pâté

Wheat/gluten-free   Dairy-free

The aubergine (eggplant) in this recipe makes a good substitute for breadcrumbs as a 'thickener', although it will make for a softer-textured pâté. You should not need any extra salt as the smoked fish itself, the lemon juice and the pepper will give lots of flavour.

Ingredients

SERVES 4

METRIC (IMPERIAL)	AMERICAN
1 medium aubergine (eggplant), sliced thickly	1 medium
2 cloves garlic, peeled	2 cloves
200g (7oz) smoked trout, mackerel or salmon, skin and any bones removed	7oz
juice of 1 small lemon	juice of 1 small
freshly ground black pepper	

Method

1 Steam the aubergine (eggplant) and garlic cloves until both are quite soft. Carefully remove skin from the aubergine (eggplant).
2 Purée the fish in a food processor with the garlic and aubergine (eggplant).
3 Season to taste with lemon juice and black pepper.
4 Serve with wheat/gluten-free toast or crackers or with a salad.

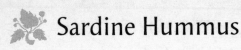

Sardine Hummus

Wheat/gluten-free 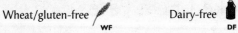 Dairy-free
WF   DF

This delicious variation on standard hummus is high in fibre and includes lots of oily fish.

Ingredients

SERVES 4

METRIC (IMPERIAL)	AMERICAN
2 x 420g (14oz) tins chickpeas (garbanzos), drained	2 x 14oz
3–4 cloves garlic, peeled	3–4 cloves
½ teaspoon ground cumin	½ teaspoon
2 x 120g (4oz) tins whole sardines in oil	2 x 4oz
juice of 2 lemons	juice of 2
sea salt and freshly ground black pepper	
2 tablespoons fresh parsley, chopped finely (optional)	2 tablespoons

Method

1 Put the chickpeas (garbanzos), garlic, ground cumin and sardines with their oil in a food processor and purée until the hummus is as smooth as you want it.
2 Add lemon juice, salt and pepper to taste and the chopped parsley, if desired.
3 Serve with crudités, wheat- and gluten-free pitta bread or toast or rice cakes.

Avocado and Strawberry Surprise

Wheat/gluten-free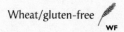

This summery and pretty mixture is high in vitamin E and 'good' fats, and has a moderate fibre content.

Ingredients

SERVES 4

METRIC (IMPERIAL)	AMERICAN
2 ripe avocados	2
2 tablespoons plain, creamy yoghurt	2 tablespoons
juice of 2 lemons	juice of 2
salt and freshly ground black pepper	
approx. 12 strawberries	approx. 12
4 fresh mint leaves (optional)	4

Method

1 Remove the flesh from the avocados and mash it thoroughly.
2 Add the yoghurt and some of the lemon juice with a little salt and pepper.
3 Chop the strawberries fairly small, leaving two for decoration, and mix them into the avocado purée. Taste the mixture and add more lemon juice and seasoning if necessary.
4 Spoon the mixture into ramekin dishes or glasses and chill thoroughly.
5 Just before serving, decorate each with the remaining strawberries, halved, or with a fresh mint leaf.

Avocado and Melon Salad

Wheat/gluten-free 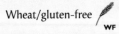 **WF**   Dairy-free **DF**

A really light and refreshing starter.

Ingredients

SERVES 4

METRIC (IMPERIAL)	**AMERICAN**
juice of 1–2 lemons	juice of 1–2
3 tablespoons olive, hazelnut or walnut oil	3 tablespoons
8 fresh mint leaves, chopped roughly	8
sea salt and freshly ground black pepper	
2 medium ripe avocados, peeled and sliced	2 medium
1 small cantaloupe melon[1], diced	1 small

Method

1 Mix the lemon juice, oil and mint leaves and season to taste with salt and pepper.
2 Add the avocado slices and diced melon and toss well but gently.
3 Leave to marinate for a couple of hours at room temperature before serving in glass dishes.

[1] If you cannot get cantaloupe, an Ogen or Galia will do, or even a honeydew.

CHAPTER 12

Fish dishes

Smoked Haddock Chowder

Wheat/gluten-free 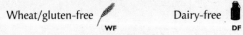 **WF**   Dairy-free **DF**

Low in fat and relatively high in fibre, this is a really filling winter main-course soup. If possible, make it a day in advance to give the flavours time to mature. Seaweeds can be purchased from health-food stores or upmarket delis.

Ingredients

SERVES 4

METRIC (IMPERIAL)	AMERICAN
1 medium leek, trimmed and sliced	1 medium
100g (4oz) small new potatoes, halved or sliced	4oz
75g (3oz) celeriac, cut into small cubes	3oz
2 cloves garlic, peeled and sliced	2 cloves
½ lemon, sliced	½
1.5 litres (2½ pints) water	6¼ cups
120ml (4fl oz) dry white wine	½ cup
200g (7oz) smoked haddock fillets, skinned and cut into pieces	7oz
2 fresh tomatoes, skinned and chopped	2
2 handfuls dried, mixed seaweeds	2 handfuls
sea salt and freshly ground black pepper	

Method

1 Put the leek, potatoes, celeriac, garlic and lemon in a wide pan with 1 litre (1¾ pints) of water and the wine.

2 Bring to the boil and simmer briskly, uncovered, for 20–30 minutes or until the vegetables are cooked.

3 Add the smoked haddock and tomatoes and cook for a further 10 minutes. The liquid should be quite reduced.

4 Add the remaining water plus the seaweeds, bring back to the boil and continue to cook for a further 15 minutes.

5 Season to taste, if necessary, before serving.

Smoked Mackerel and Bean Salad

Wheat/gluten-free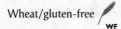

Dairy-free

You could also make this salad with tinned sardines or tuna, if you were avoiding smoked foods. In that case, you might need to season it with a little salt as well. The beans and butterbeans make this a fairly high-fibre dish.

Ingredients

SERVES 4

METRIC (IMPERIAL)	AMERICAN
400g (14oz) fresh runner beans, trimmed	14oz
1 x 425g (15oz) tin of butterbeans, drained	1 x 15oz
10 spring onions (scallions), trimmed and chopped	10
2 smoked mackerel fillets	2
juice of 1 lemon	juice of 1
freshly ground black pepper	
chopped parsley	

Method

1 Slice the runner beans into fairly small pieces and steam over boiling water for 5–6 minutes or until they are just beginning to soften but have not lost their colour or all their 'crunch'.

2 While still warm, mix the runner beans in a big bowl with the butterbeans and the chopped spring onions (scallions).

3 Break the fish into small pieces with your hands, making sure to remove all skin and bones, and mix it in.

4 Season to taste with lemon juice and black pepper. Spoon the salad into a dish and sprinkle with chopped parsley before serving.

Halibut with Leeks, Spinach and Courgettes (Small Zucchini)

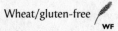 Wheat/gluten-free Dairy-free

WF

DF

You can use any white fish in this recipe. Very low fat and relatively low in fibre, this recipe has the advantage of coming complete with its vegetables.

Ingredients

SERVES 4

METRIC (IMPERIAL)	AMERICAN
Fish	
3 tablespoons olive oil	3 tablespoons
4 medium leeks, trimmed and sliced thinly	4 medium
4 fillets halibut or other white fish	4 fillets
8 slices lemon	8 slices
approx. 200ml (7fl oz) fish stock, water or white wine and water mixed	⅞ cup
handful fresh coriander, chopped roughly	handful
Vegetables	
4 tablespoons olive oil	4 tablespoons
2 medium leeks, trimmed and sliced thinly	2 medium
4 courgettes (small zucchini), wiped and sliced fairly thinly	4
200g (7oz) green beans, topped, tailed and cut in half	7oz
250g (9oz) fresh, washed spinach, well drained	9oz
sea salt and freshly ground black pepper	

Method

Fish

1 Heat the oil in a wide pan and gently sweat the leeks for 10–15 minutes or until quite soft.

2 Lay the fish fillets over the leeks, top with the lemon slices and add the fish stock or other liquid. Cover the pan and continue to cook gently for a further 15 minutes or until the fish is cooked through.

Vegetables

1 Heat the oil in a deep pan and add the leeks and courgettes (small zucchini). Cover and cook gently for 10 minutes.

2 Add the green beans and the spinach. Re-cover the pan and continue to cook for a further 10 minutes, by which time the beans should still be slightly *al dente* and the spinach cooked.

3 Season lightly with salt and pepper.

To serve

Discard the lemon slices and carefully move the fish on its bed of leeks onto a warmed serving dish. Surround with (or serve accompanied by if the serving dish is not big enough) the vegetables. Sprinkle the chopped coriander over the fish just before serving.

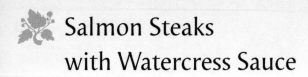

Salmon Steaks with Watercress Sauce

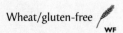

Wheat/gluten-free
WF

A delicious, low-fibre fish dish with a delicate flavour.

Ingredients
SERVES 4

METRIC (IMPERIAL)	AMERICAN
4 salmon steaks	4
1 lemon, sliced	1
3 sprigs parsley	3 sprigs
½ bulb fennel, sliced	½ bulb
4 tablespoons olive oil	4 tablespoons
2 small cloves garlic, peeled and sliced	2 small cloves
4 spring onions (scallions), trimmed and sliced	4
4 tablespoons long-grain rice	4 tablespoons
8 cardamom pods, bruised with a rolling pin	8
juice of ½ lemon	juice of ½
2 stalks parsley, trimmed and finely chopped	2 stalks
115g (4oz) watercress	4oz
140g (5oz) plain mild yoghurt	5oz
2 tablespoons cooking juices	2 tablespoons

Method

1   Lay the salmon steaks in a large pan with the lemon, parsley and fennel, and cover with water. Bring slowly to the boil, and as soon as the water boils, turn off the heat. Leave the salmon to cook and cool in the liquid.

2   When the fish is cold, remove it and reserve the liquid, setting aside 2 tablespoons for the sauce.

3   Heat the oil in a heavy pan and gently cook the garlic and spring onions (scallions) for a few minutes.

4   Add the rice and cardamom pods and cover with the fish cooking liquid. Bring slowly to the boil and simmer until the rice is cooked, adding extra water if needed. When cooked, add lemon juice to taste and stir in the parsley.

5   Meanwhile, purée the watercress in a food processor with the yoghurt. Thin with the fish stock.

6   To serve, spread the rice out on a serving dish, lay the salmon steaks on the rice and spoon the watercress sauce over the top. The whole dish should be served warm or at room temperature.

Tuna, Anchovy and Pasta Pie

Wheat/gluten-free 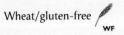 Dairy-free

WF   DF

There are now a number of excellent wheat- and/or gluten-free pastas, both fresh and dried, to be found in health-foods stores, some supermarkets or by mail order. This is a relatively low-fibre dish.

Ingredients   SERVES 4

METRIC (IMPERIAL)	AMERICAN
225g (8oz) dried gluten/wheat-free pasta shapes	8oz
1 x 50g (2oz) tin of anchovies	1 x 2oz
1 x 185g (6oz) tin of tuna in oil	1 x 6oz
4 tablespoons oil from the anchovy and tuna tins	4 tablespoons
1 large onion, chopped finely	1 large
100g (4oz) mushrooms, sliced	4oz
1 heaped tablespoon potato flour	1 heaped tablespoon
600ml (1 pint) soya milk, fish or vegetable stock or a combination of stock and white wine	2½ cups
50g (2oz) fresh or frozen petits pois	2oz
juice of 1 lemon	juice of 1
freshly ground black pepper	
1 small packet plain potato crisps, crushed	1 small packet

Method

1 Cook the pasta in plenty of fast-boiling water, following the instructions on the packet. Keep it warm.

2 Heat the oil from the fish in a pan, add the onions and mushrooms and cook gently for 10–25 minutes or until the vegetables are soft.

3 Add the potato flour, stir well, then gradually add the liquid. Bring to the boil and simmer until the sauce thickens.

4 Add 4 anchovies, chopped small, the tuna fish and the petits pois.

5 Add the cooked pasta. Mix well and season to taste with lemon juice and black pepper.

6 Turn the mixture into a pie dish, and sprinkle the crisps over the top.

7 Toast lightly under the grill before serving with a green vegetable or salad.

Stir-fried Tuna with Fennel and Artichokes

Wheat/gluten-free
WF

Dairy-free
DF

A quick and spicy, high-fibre dish with a distinctly Chinese flavour. If you are on a wheat-free diet, take care only to use tamari, as most other soy sauces contain wheat.

Ingredients

METRIC (IMPERIAL)	AMERICAN
3 tablespoons sunflower or rice oil	3 tablespoons
3 fresh green chillies, carefully seeded and sliced finely	3
3 large cloves garlic, peeled and sliced thinly	3 large cloves
6 spring onions (scallions), trimmed and chopped	6
25g (1oz) knob fresh ginger, peeled and cut into very fine matchsticks	1oz knob
1 red pepper, deseeded and sliced thinly	1
400g (14oz) Jerusalem artichokes, scrubbed, trimmed and sliced into thin matchsticks	14oz
140g (5oz) fennel, trimmed and sliced thinly	5oz
350g (12oz) fresh tuna, cubed[1]	12oz
50g (2oz) pine nuts	2oz
tamari to taste	
black pepper	
large handful fresh coriander, chopped	large handful

Method

1 Heat the oil in a wide pan or wok and briskly cook the chillies, garlic, spring onions (scallions), ginger and red pepper for 3 minutes.

2 Add the artichoke, fennel and fresh tuna, and continue to cook briskly for a further 3–5 minutes or until the tuna is cooked and the vegetables are softening but still have some crispness. If using tinned tuna, do not add it until the artichoke and fennel have been cooking for 3 minutes.

3 Add the pine nuts and season to taste with tamari and black pepper. Serve at once, sprinkled with lots of coriander.

¹ If you cannot get fresh tuna you can use 2 x 185g (6½oz) tins tuna in oil, drained and flaked.

Spaghetti with Smoked Salmon and Fromage Frais

Wheat/gluten-free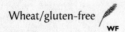

WF

This low-fibre recipe can be quite economical if you use the smoked salmon offcuts that are now available in most supermarkets. You can get gluten- and wheat-free spaghetti in a number of supermarkets and health-food stores or by mail order (see page 230).

Ingredients

SERVES 4

METRIC (IMPERIAL)	AMERICAN
100g (4oz) courgettes (small zucchini)	4oz
30ml (1fl oz) sunflower oil	⅛ cup
100g (4oz) button mushrooms, sliced finely	4oz
250ml (9fl oz) dry white wine	1⅛ cups
1 heaped teaspoon fresh dill, chopped *or*	1 heaped teaspoon
1 level teaspoon dried dill	1 level teaspoon
300g (10oz) fromage frais	10oz
225g (8oz) smoked salmon, cut in thin matchsticks	8oz
freshly ground black pepper	
juice of 1 lemon	juice of 1
340g (12oz) gluten/wheat-free spaghetti	12oz

Method

1 Wipe the courgettes (small zucchini) and cut into thin matchsticks.
2 Heat the oil in a wide pan and gently fry the mushrooms and courgettes (small zucchini) for 4–5 minutes, without letting them colour.
3 If you are using dried dill, add it at this point.
4 Add the wine, increase the heat and cook fast for a further 5 minutes to reduce the liquid.
5 Add the fresh dill and the fromage frais, and heat gently to melt the fromage frais. Add the salmon and reheat gently, but do not boil.
6 Season to taste with pepper and lemon juice. Cover, set aside and keep just warm.
7 Cook the pasta according to the instructions on the packet until just *al dente*. Drain and rinse thoroughly with boiling water.
8 Turn the pasta into a warmed serving dish and gently mix in the salmon in its sauce before serving.

Salmon, Apple and Peanut Salad

Wheat/gluten-free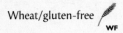
WF

The combination of crunchy apples and peanuts with the softness of the salmon gives this salad a great texture. The nuts and raw apple make this a relatively high-fibre dish.

Ingredients

SERVES 4

METRIC (IMPERIAL)	AMERICAN
340g (12oz) salmon fillet	12oz
2 medium-sized tart eating apples	2 medium-sized
85g (3oz) dry roasted peanuts	3oz
120ml (4fl oz) plain Greek yoghurt	½ cup
juice of ½ a large lemon	juice of ½ a large
freshly ground black pepper	
1 head crisp lettuce, chopped roughly	1 head

Method

1. Cook the salmon. You can grill dribbled with a little oil, steam over water with several slices of lemon, or microwave in 25cm (1 inch) of water with a few slices of lemon. Drain and flake into largish chunks.
2. Core and dice the apples but do not peel, and mix with the salmon and peanuts.
3. Season and thin the yoghurt with the lemon juice and pepper – you should not need any extra salt as the peanuts will be salted.
4. Gently toss the fish and apple mixture in the yoghurt, and adjust the seasoning to taste.
5. Arrange the lettuce on a serving dish and pile the fish mixture on top to serve.

CHAPTER 13

Meat and poultry dishes

Tajine of Beef with Okra

Wheat/gluten-free 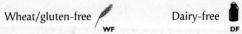   Dairy-free

WF   **DF**

This recipe is based on a North African beef dish which would normally be served with couscous. If you are on a wheat-free diet, you could serve it with quinoa (the South American grain) or rice and a fresh green salad. In either case, it will be a relatively low-fibre dish.

Ingredients

SERVES 4

METRIC (IMPERIAL)	AMERICAN
4 tablespoons olive oil	4 tablespoons
2 medium onions, peeled and sliced finely	2 medium
2 cloves garlic, peeled and sliced finely	2 cloves
170g (6oz) fresh okra[1], topped and tailed and halved if very big	6oz
600g (22oz) stewing or braising beef	22oz
2 teaspoons tomato purée (paste)	2 teaspoons
1 teaspoon ground cumin	1 teaspoon
4 fresh tomatoes, skinned[2], then chopped into small dice	4
200ml (7fl oz) water	⅞ cup
salt and pepper	

Method

1 Heat the oil in a heavy pan and add the onions, garlic and fresh okra. Cook together briskly for 3–4 minutes.
2 Add the beef, the tomato purée (paste), cumin and diced tomato and continue to cook briskly for another 3–4 minutes.
3 Add the water and a little salt and pepper. Bring back to the boil then turn the heat down low and simmer gently for 1½–2 hours, or until the meat is very tender.
4 Adjust the seasoning to taste.

[1] If you cannot get fresh okra you can use 100g (4oz) tinned or bottled okra.
[2] Drop into a bowl of boiling water for 3–4 minutes then cool under a cold tap. The skin should then peel off easily.

Slow-cook Beef with Garlic

Wheat/gluten-free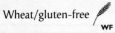
WF

Dairy-free
DF

The flavour of this dish comes out best if it is cooked very, very slowly – a slow cooker overnight is ideal. If you need it to be very low in fibre, cook the beef with the vegetables so it takes on their flavour but leave the turnips out when you serve it.

Ingredients

SERVES 4

METRIC (IMPERIAL)	AMERICAN
8 cloves garlic, peeled and left whole	8
550g (1¼lb) approx. joint of topside or other braising beef	1¼lb
4 turnips, peeled and left whole	4
1 medium leek, trimmed and sliced thickly	1 medium
1 x 50g (2oz) piece fresh ginger, peeled and left whole (optional)	1 x 2oz piece
3 bay leaves	3
1 bouquet garni	1
8 black peppercorns, bruised with a rolling pin	8
500ml (18fl oz) water	2¼ cups
2 teaspoons potato flour	2 teaspoons
sea salt	
handful fresh parsley or coriander	handful

Method

1 Put the garlic, beef, turnips, leek, whole piece of ginger, dried herbs, peppercorns and water in a heavy, lidded pot.

2 Bring slowly to the boil and cook very slowly for 3–4 hours or overnight in a slow cooker.

3 Remove the piece of ginger.

4 Mix the potato flour with 2 tablespoons of the cooking juices and return to the pot. Bring back to a simmer and cook gently to thicken.

5 Season to taste with sea salt and further ground black pepper if required, and add the freshly chopped parsley or coriander just before serving.

Lentils with Carrots and Sausages

May be wheat/gluten-free

The flavour of this excellent winter dish comes out best if you cook it the day before you want to eat it. The root vegetables and lentils make it a high-fibre dish, and if you are on either a wheat/gluten- or a dairy-free diet, you need to examine your sausages carefully. Frankfurters are normally wheat/gluten-free but do contain dairy products; regular 'English' sausages normally contain wheat/gluten, although it is now possible to buy gluten-free sausages.

Ingredients

SERVES 4

METRIC (IMPERIAL)	AMERICAN
2 large carrots, scrubbed and halved	2 large
4 small onions, peeled and left whole	4 small
4 large frankfurters or regular sausages (*see above*)	4 large
6 tablespoons brown or Puy lentils	6 tablespoons
4 tablespoons red lentils	4 tablespoons
1 litre (1¾ pints) water or gluten/ wheat-free vegetable stock	4¼ cups
12 coriander seeds, bruised with a rolling pin	12
sea salt and freshly ground black pepper	
handful parsley, chopped	handful

Method

1 Put all the ingredients apart from the parsley in a heavy, deep pan and bring slowly to the boil. Cover and simmer gently for 30 minutes.

2 Remove the lid and simmer briskly until most of the liquid has been absorbed and the red lentils have dissolved into a purée.

3 If you have time, cool and leave for 24 hours before reheating. To serve, reheat, adjust the seasoning to taste and stir in the chopped parsley.

Leg of Lamb with Butterbeans and Artichokes

Wheat/gluten-free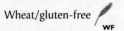
WF

Dairy-free
DF

A really delicious and easy way to cook lamb, this dish is high in fibre because of the butterbeans. It should not need any further seasoning because the casserole cooking will bring out the flavour of the herbs.

Ingredients

SERVES 4

METRIC (IMPERIAL)	AMERICAN
1 smallish leg lamb (approx. 1.8 kg/4lb)	1 smallish (approx. 4lb)
6 large cloves garlic, peeled	6 large
2 leeks, sliced thickly	2
2 tablespoons olive oil	2 tablespoons
2 sprigs fresh rosemary *or*	2 sprigs
2 teaspoons dried rosemary	2 teaspoons
3 bay leaves	3
550g (1¼lb) tinned butterbeans, drained	1¼lb
285g (10oz) tinned or frozen artichoke hearts	10oz

Method

1 Heat the oven to 180°C/350°F/Gas Mark 4.

2 Cut 4–6 slashes in the lamb and insert halved cloves of garlic into each.

3 Put the sliced leeks with the rest of the garlic and the oil in a heavy casserole, large enough to hold the lamb. Lay the rosemary and bay leaves over the vegetables and place the lamb on top. Cover and bake for 1 hour.

4 Remove the casserole from the oven. Transfer the lamb to a baking tray and return to the oven for a further half hour to brown the outside.

5 Add the drained butterbeans and the artichoke hearts with some of their juice (but not if they have been canned in any kind of vinegar) to the vegetables in the casserole and mix together.

6 Return the lamb to the casserole, re-cover and cook for a further 20–30 minutes to allow the flavours to amalgamate.

7 Serve with plenty of green and root vegetables – and, when you are finished, keep the bone to make soup!

Roast Lamb
with Mushroom Cream Sauce

Wheat/gluten-free 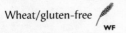 **WF**   Dairy-free **DF**

Ingredients   SERVES 4

METRIC (IMPERIAL)	AMERICAN
750g (1½lb) boned and rolled leg or shoulder of lamb	1½lb
sprig fresh rosemary *or*	sprig
½ teaspoon dried rosemary	½ teaspoon
2 tablespoons virgin olive or sunflower oil	2 tablespoons
1 small onion, chopped finely	1 small
100g (4oz) button mushrooms, stems removed and sliced thinly	4oz
1 small cooking (or sharp eating) apple, peeled, cored and chopped finely	1 small
½ level tablespoon cornflour (cornstarch)	½ level tablespoon
250ml (8fl oz) gluten/wheat-free vegetable or chicken stock	1 cup
60ml (2fl oz) soya cream	¼ cup
1–2 tablespoons good quality French mustard (check ingredients)	1–2 tablespoons
salt and pepper	

Method

1 Sit the lamb on top of the rosemary in a baking tray and bake in a moderate oven (170°C/325°F/Gas Mark 3) for 1 hour and 20 minutes.

2 Meanwhile, heat the oil in a heavy pan and gently cook the onions with the mushrooms and apple until quite soft.

3 Add the cornflour (cornstarch), stir around for a couple of minutes, then gradually add the stock. Bring back to a simmer and cook for a few minutes, stirring all the while, until the sauce thickens slightly.

4 Add the soya cream and 1 tablespoon of the mustard. Taste for flavour and add more mustard, salt or pepper to suit your palate. Set aside until the lamb is cooked.

5 Just before serving, pour the juices from the lamb into the sauce and reheat to a simmer. Pour the sauce into a preheated flatish serving dish, cut the strings from the lamb and place in the middle of the sauce to serve.

Red Chicken with Chilli

Wheat/gluten-free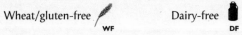
WF

Dairy-free
DF

A very colourful and tasty dish with a moderate amount of fibre and lots of flavour.

Ingredients

SERVES 4

METRIC (IMPERIAL)	AMERICAN
2 tablespoons olive oil	2 tablespoons
1 teaspoon cayenne pepper	1 teaspoon
1–2 red chillies (depending on how hot you want it), seeds and pith removed, sliced thinly	1–2
4 cloves garlic, sliced	4
2 medium red peppers, sliced	2 medium
1 chicken, jointed	1
400g (14oz) can chopped tomatoes	14oz
8 cardamom seeds	8
1 scant teaspoon each sea salt and black peppercorns	1 scant teaspoon each
4 bay leaves	4
4 tablespoons white rice	4 tablespoons
350ml (12fl oz) water	1½ cups
juice of 1–2 lemons	juice of 1–2
6 spring onions (scallions), chopped	6

Method

1 Heat the oil in a deep pan, add the cayenne, chillies, garlic and red peppers, cover and cook gently for 15 minutes or until the peppers are quite soft.

2 Add the chicken joints, tomatoes, cardamom seeds and seasoning, cover the pan once more and continue to cook gently for a further 30 minutes.

3 Add the rice and water, stir well and bring to the boil. Simmer uncovered for a further 15 minutes or until the rice is cooked. Add a little extra water if needed.

4 Season to taste with lemon juice and sprinkle over the chopped spring onions (scallions). Serve warm or at room temperature with a green salad.

Lamb Chops with Black Olives

Wheat/gluten-free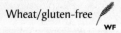
WF

Dairy-free
DF

The olives give this dish lots of flavour so you should not need any extra salt. This is a good dish for those on low-fibre diets.

Ingredients

SERVES 4

METRIC (IMPERIAL)	AMERICAN
3 tablespoons virgin olive or sunflower oil	3 tablespoons
8 shoulder lamb chops	8
3 cloves garlic, minced	3
500ml (18fl oz) dry white wine	2¼ cups
4 tablespoons tomato purée (paste)	4 tablespoons
14 calamata olives, pitted	14
4 teaspoons fresh rosemary	4 teaspoons
salt and pepper to taste	

Method

1 Heat the oil in a deep pan. Brown the chops on both sides and remove from the pan.

2 Sauté the minced garlic for 1 minute. Add the white wine and tomato purée and whisk until blended.

3 Add the olives and rosemary (about 1 tsp each initially).

4 Return the chops to the pan and bring the liquid to the boil, reduce to a simmer and cook, covered, for 1 hour. Turn chops about every 20 minutes.

5 Cool, cover and refrigerate overnight. Reheat, adjust the seasoning to taste, and serve with lots of boiled rice.

Breast of Chicken Dauphinoise

Wheat/gluten-free 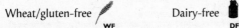 **WF**   Dairy-free **DF**

This relatively low-fibre dish is a tasty and easy way to cook chicken breasts, and keeps them very moist.

Ingredients

SERVES 4

METRIC (IMPERIAL)	AMERICAN
6 tablespoons olive oil	6 tablespoons
8 medium waxy potatoes, scrubbed	8 medium
2 medium onions, peeled and sliced very thinly	2 medium
4 large cloves garlic, peeled and sliced very thinly	4 large
4 chicken breasts, skins removed	4
4 tablespoons plain fromage frais	4 tablespoons
sea salt and freshly ground black pepper	

Method

1 Heat the oven to 180°C/350°F/Gas Mark 4.
2 Pour 4 tablespoons of the oil into an oven-proof casserole large enough to hold all the ingredients.
3 Slice half the potatoes very thinly and lay them out on the bottom of the casserole. Cover with the onions, the garlic and then the chicken breasts.
4 Spread the fromage frais over the chicken breasts, season with sea salt and black pepper, then cover with the rest of the potatoes, sliced very thinly.
5 Brush the top of the potatoes with the remaining oil, cover the dish and bake for 35 minutes.
6 Remove the lid and continue to bake for a further 15–20 minutes to brown the top of the potatoes.
7 Serve at once with a green vegetable.

Risotto with Chicken and Lemon

Wheat/gluten-free **WF**　　　Dairy-free **DF**

A pretty, green and white, low-fibre salad – ideal for a summer lunch or picnic.

Ingredients

SERVES 4

METRIC (IMPERIAL)	AMERICAN
4 tablespoons olive oil *with*	4 tablespoons
2 tablespoons water	2 tablespoons
2 small onions, peeled and chopped finely	2 small
2 large cloves garlic, peeled and chopped	2 large
6 tablespoons long-grain white rice	6 tablespoons
600ml (1 pint) vegetable stock (check ingredients)	2½ cups
150g (6oz) cooked chicken or turkey, cut into small pieces	6oz
6 spring onions (scallions), trimmed and chopped fairly small	6
juice of 1 lemon	juice of 1
¼ teaspoon salt	¼ teaspoon

Method

1　Put the oil and water into a wide pan with the onions and garlic. Cook very gently for 5 minutes or until the onion is just softening.
2　Add the rice, stir around for a few minutes, then add the stock.
3　Bring to the boil, cover and simmer gently for 20–30 minutes or until the liquid is absorbed and the rice quite cooked. If necessary, add a little extra water.
4　Add the chicken or turkey, spring onions and lemon juice, and season to taste with salt.
5　Serve warm or at room temperature, alone or with a mixed green salad.

Cold Chicken
with Creamy Green Sauce

Wheat/gluten-free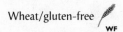

*The flavour of this fresh-tasting, medium-fibre dish will change accord-
ing to the herbs you use. Choose whatever you fancy or have available in
the garden, perhaps mint, basil or savoury.*

Ingredients

SERVES 4

METRIC (IMPERIAL)	AMERICAN
225g (8oz) courgettes (small zucchini), sliced	8oz
150g (6oz) broccoli florets	6oz
small bunch fresh herbs	small bunch
4 tablespoons plain yoghurt	4 tablespoons
salt and pepper	
450g (1lb) cooked chicken meat, sliced	1lb
225g (8oz) button mushrooms, sliced	8oz

Method

1 Steam the courgettes (small zucchini) and broccoli until quite soft.
   Reserve the cooking water.
2 Put the vegetables in a food processor or liquidizer (blender) with the
   herbs and yoghurt and process until they make a fairly smooth purée.
   If you want the sauce to be totally smooth, you will need to rub the
   purée through a sieve as well.
3 Season to taste with salt and pepper and thin with a few tablespoons
   of the cooking water.
4 To serve, lay the chicken in a dish and cover with the raw sliced
   mushrooms, then spoon over the sauce. Decorate with watercress or
   a few more chopped herbs.

Roast Chicken with Sweet Potatoes and Onions

Wheat/gluten-free 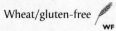 **WF**   Dairy-free **DF**

This simple dish is high in vitamins C and E and has a moderate fibre content. Slow cooking should produce the most delicious juices in the bottom of the roasting pan, which will need no further adornment.

Ingredients
SERVES 4

METRIC (IMPERIAL)	AMERICAN
1 medium chicken	1 medium
4 large sweet potatoes, peeled and halved	4 large
4 medium onions, peeled and left whole	4 medium
4 baby onions or shallots, peeled and left whole	4
8 cloves garlic, peeled and left whole	8
4 tablespoons olive oil	4 tablespoons
8 bacon rashers (slices)	8

Method

1 Heat the oven to 180°C/350°F/Gas Mark 4.
2 Put the chicken in a large roasting dish and surround it with the vegetables and garlic. Pour over the oil and roll the vegetables in it, making sure they are coated all over.
3 Lay the bacon rashers over the breast and legs of the chicken and cover with a sheet of aluminium foil.
4 Bake for 1–1½ hours or until the juices run clear from the chicken. Every half an hour, turn the vegetables to make sure they are cooking evenly. Remove the foil for the last 30 minutes to allow the chicken and bacon to brown.
5 To serve, place the chicken in a warmed serving dish, surround with the vegetables and spoon over all the juices from the baking dish.
6 Serve with green vegetables or a green salad.

CHAPTER 14

Light lunches, salads and vegetarian dishes

Fresh Herb Frittata

Wheat/gluten-free 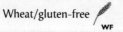 **WF**

Dairy-free **DF**

This omelette (omelet) is perfect for the summer when herbs are fresh. It can be eaten warm or left to cool and eaten in wedges, or serve with a salad for a picnic.

Ingredients

SERVES 4

METRIC (IMPERIAL)	AMERICAN
3 tablespoons olive oil	3 tablespoons
1 medium leek, sliced very finely	1 medium
2 cloves garlic, peeled and sliced	2
40g (1½oz) fresh broad (fava) beans (optional)	1½oz
1 handful fresh spinach	1 handful
1 handful fresh watercress	1 handful
2 sprigs fresh mint	2 sprigs
1 handful fresh parsley	1 handful
4 sprigs fresh coriander (optional)	4 sprigs
7 medium eggs	7 medium
2 tablespoons water	2 tablespoons
1 tablespoon pine nuts	1 tablespoon
sea salt and freshly ground black pepper	

Method

1 Heat 2 tablespoons of the oil and very gently cook the leeks and garlic until quite soft.

2 Meanwhile, steam the broad (fava) beans, if using, until just cooked. Chop the spinach and all the herbs roughly.

3 Beat the eggs with the water in a large bowl. Add the leeks and garlic, the beans, chopped spinach and herbs and pine nuts. Season generously.

4 Heat the remaining tablespoon of olive oil in a wide pan until almost smoking. Pour in the egg mixture and cook briskly for a couple of minutes until the bottom of the omelette (omelet) is firm. Place under a hot grill to cook the top.

5 Alternatively, pour the mixture into a wide ovenproof dish and cook in a medium oven (180°C/350°F/Gas Mark 4) for 30–40 minutes or until firm.

6 Serve warm or at room temperature with a salad or crackers.

Quiche Primavera

May be wheat/gluten-free
WF

Dairy-free
DF

A dairy-free quiche for which you can use a proprietary wheat-free pastry mix or the recipe on page 175.

Ingredients

SERVES 4

METRIC (IMPERIAL)	AMERICAN
450g (1lb) tomatoes	1lb
1 onion, chopped finely	1
2 tablespoons olive or sunflower oil	2 tablespoons
6 spring onions (scallions), chopped finely	6
100g (4oz) mushrooms, sliced	4oz
150g (6oz) broccoli florets	6oz
20-cm (8-inch) pastry shell, baked blind	8-inch
1 bunch watercress, chopped	1 bunch
4 eggs	4
150ml (5fl oz) white wine	⅝ cup
salt and pepper	

Method

1 Chop the tomatoes roughly and put them in a pan with the onion.

2 Cover the pan, bring to the boil and simmer briskly for 30 minutes or until the tomatoes are quite mushy. Purée in a food processor or liquidizer, strain out the pips and make it up to 300ml/10fl oz/2¼ cups with water.

3 Meanwhile, heat the oil in a heavy pan and gently cook the spring onions (scallions) for a few minutes. Add the mushrooms and cook rather more briskly for another couple of minutes.

4 Steam the broccoli florets for 5 minutes or until just softening, then remove them from the heat.

5 Arrange the broccoli and mushroom/onion mixture in the bottom of the pastry shell.

6 Mix the chopped watercress with the eggs, the tomato sauce and the wine, and season generously. Pour over the vegetables in the pastry shell.

7 Bake for 30–45 minutes in a moderately cool oven (150°C/300°F/Gas Mark 2) or until the flan is set and lightly browned.

Farfalle with Spinach and Pumpkin Sauce

Wheat/gluten-free **WF**   Dairy-free **DF**

Gluten- and wheat-free pastas are fairly easy to find in health-food stores and some supermarkets or via mail order (see page 230). Pumpkin oil is to be found in many delicatessens and has a wonderful rich, smoky flavour. This is a relatively high-fibre dish because of the seeds and nuts.

Ingredients   SERVES 4

METRIC (IMPERIAL)	AMERICAN
8 tablespoons olive oil	8 tablespoons
2 tablespoons water	2 tablespoons
400g (14oz) mixed mushrooms, sliced	14oz
100g (4oz) fresh spinach, chopped	4oz
2 tablespoons pine nuts	2 tablespoons
2 tablespoons pumpkin oil	2 tablespoons
juice of 1 lemon	juice of 1
300g (10oz) wheat/gluten-free farfalle or other pasta	10oz

Method

Sauce

1 Gently heat the oil with the water.
2 Add the mushrooms and spinach and cook fairly briskly for 5 minutes or until the spinach leaves have wilted.
3 Add the pine nuts, cook for another minute or two, then season with the pumpkin oil and lemon juice.

Pasta

1 Cook the pasta in plenty of fast-boiling water according to the instructions on the packet.
2 Drain, toss in a little olive oil, pile onto four plates and spoon over the sauce.
3 Serve at once.

Pasta with Cabbage

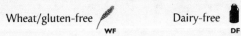

Wheat/gluten-free **WF**   Dairy-free **DF**

This unusual combination works well both in gastronomic and health terms. You can easily convert it from a vegetarian to a meat dish by adding chopped ham or bacon to the cabbage mix. It is a fairly high-fibre recipe.

Ingredients

SERVES 4

METRIC (IMPERIAL)	AMERICAN
4 tablespoons olive or sunflower oil	4 tablespoons
2 medium onions, peeled and chopped roughly	2 medium
4 bacon rashers (slices), chopped up (optional)	4
225g (8oz) white cabbage, chopped roughly	8oz
225g (8oz) Brussels sprouts, halved	8oz
2 teaspoons caraway seeds	2 teaspoons
1 tsp dried dill	1 tsp
300ml (10fl oz) vegetable stock (check ingredients)	1¼ cups
salt and pepper	
170g (6oz) wheat/gluten-free pasta shapes	6oz
2 thick slices lean ham (optional)	2

Method

1 Heat the oil in a large pan and gently fry the onions and bacon (if using) until the onions are just soft and lightly tanned.

2 Add the cabbage and Brussels sprouts and continue to cook for a few minutes, then add the caraway seeds, dill, stock and a little seasoning.

3 Cover and simmer for 5–10 minutes or until the cabbage is cooked but still slightly crunchy.

4 Meanwhile, cook the pasta in fast-boiling water till just *al dente*. Drain.

5 If you are using the ham, dice finely and mix into the cabbage along with the pasta.

6 Adjust seasoning to taste and serve at once.

Wheat-free Gnocchi with Courgettes (Small Zucchini) and Mushrooms

Wheat/gluten-free ✎ **WF**   Dairy-free **DF**

Gnocchi are often off the menu for those on a wheat/gluten-free diet, but in fact they work very well using potatoes.

Ingredients   SERVES 4

METRIC (IMPERIAL)	AMERICAN
Gnocchi	
1 kg (2¼lb) floury, baking-type potatoes	2¼lb
1 egg, beaten	1
1 teaspoon salt	1 teaspoon
120g (4oz) potato flour	4oz
Sauce	
4 tablespoons olive oil	4 tablespoons
2 medium courgettes (small zucchini), wiped and sliced thickly	2 medium
100g (4oz) mushrooms, sliced or halved	4oz
50g (2oz) smoked tofu, diced (optional)	2oz
50g (2oz) sprouted seeds of your choice (optional)	2oz
1 tablespoon pumpkin seeds	1 tablespoon
tamari or sea salt and black pepper to season	

Method

Gnocchi

1 Steam the potatoes in their skins until just cooked.
2 Skin them while still hot and purée in a ricer or through the small disc of a food mill, straight onto a work surface lightly floured with potato flour.
3 Spread the purée about to cool it then, gradually, add the beaten egg, the salt and most (all, if you need it) of the potato flour. Knead gently until you have a soft dough (batter) which is smooth and slightly sticky.
4 Roll the dough (batter) into 2.5cm (1-inch) sausages, then cut into 2cm (³/₄-inch) chunks. Impress a fork lightly in the middle of each gnocchi. Set aside.

Sauce

1 Heat the oil in a deep pan and add the courgettes (small zucchini), mushrooms and tofu if using.
2 Cook gently, uncovered, for 10–15 minutes or until just cooked but still slightly *al dente*. Add the sprouted seeds if using and pumpkin seeds and season to taste.

To serve

1 Bring a large pan of lightly salted water to the boil.
2 Cook the gnocchi in 3 or 4 batches, lowering each batch into the water with a slotted spoon. They will sink to the bottom so stir lightly to prevent them sticking, and very soon they will float to the top. Count slowly to 10, then remove the gnocchi with the slotted spoon and put in a heated dish with a little of the sauce. Then cook the next batch, and so on until all are done.
3 Mix the gnocchi carefully with the courgette (small zucchini) mixture and serve at once.

Rice with Smoked Tofu (Bean Curd) and Peas

Wheat/gluten-free 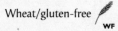 Dairy-free

This recipe is an adaptation of the classic Indian paneer with rice and peas but it works very well with plain or smoked tofu substituted for the paneer. It is quite low in fibre.

Ingredients

SERVES 4

METRIC (IMPERIAL)	AMERICAN
225g (8oz) long-grain rice	8oz
100g (4oz) plain or smoked tofu (bean curd)	4oz
4 tablespoons sunflower oil	4 tablespoons
2 bay leaves	2
2.5cm (1-inch) stick cinnamon	1-inch stick
4 whole cardamom pods	4
125g (5oz) peas, shelled fresh or defrosted frozen	5oz
1 small fresh hot green chilli pepper, sliced into fine half-rings	1 small
½ teaspoon ground cumin seeds	½ teaspoon
handful fresh flat parsley or coriander leaves	handful
sea salt and black pepper	

Method

1 Wash the rice in several changes of water, soak for 30 minutes then drain.

2 Cube the tofu (bean curd).

3 Heat the oil in a wide pan and fry the cubes of tofu quickly until coloured on two sides then remove and set aside.

4 Transfer the oil into a large pan with a well-fitting lid. Heat again, add the bay leaves, cinnamon and cardamom, rice, peas, chilli and cumin seeds. Stir and fry gently for 5 minutes.

5 Add 400ml (14fl oz) water and bring to the boil. Cover, turn the heat down very low and cook for 25 minutes. If it dries up before the rice is cooked, add a little more water.

6 Add the tofu (bean curd) pieces, cook for another few minutes then turn off the heat and leave to sit, covered, for 10 minutes.

7 Remove the bay leaves, cinnamon sticks and cardamom pods, chop and add the parsley or coriander and adjust the seasoning to taste.

8 Serve alone or with a green salad.

Spinach and Artichoke Flan

May be wheat/gluten-free
WF

Another delicious flan which can be prepared in advance and eaten warm or at room temperature. You can use a proprietary gluten/wheat-free flour mix or the pastry recipe on page 175. The seeds make this a relatively high-fibre dish but provide lots of 'good' nutrients.

Ingredients

SERVES 6

METRIC (IMPERIAL)	AMERICAN
100g (4oz) fromage frais	4oz
1 x 20cm (8-inch) flan case, ready baked	1 x 8-inch
100g (4oz) fresh leaf spinach (or frozen, defrosted and drained), cooked	4oz
50g (2oz) pumpkin seeds	2oz
100g (4oz) artichoke hearts, tinned (or frozen, defrosted and drained)	4oz
25g (1oz) sunflower seeds, lightly toasted under the grill	1oz
pumpkin oil	
freshly ground black pepper	

Method

1 Heat the oven to 180°C/350°F/Gas Mark 4.
2 Spread the fromage frais over the bottom of the flan dish.
3 Mix the spinach with the pumpkin seeds and spread over the fromage frais, then arrange the artichoke hearts on top.
4 If you want to eat the flan warm, cover with aluminium foil to stop the artichoke hearts drying out and bake for 20 minutes.
5 To serve, sprinkle over the sunflower seeds, drizzle over some pumpkin oil and grind over some black pepper.

Cauliflower with Anchovies and Lemon

Wheat/gluten-free **WF**   Dairy-free **DF**

This delicious salad is Egyptian in origin. If you want to make it totally vegetarian, you could substitute 75g (3oz) of smoked tofu (bean curd) and 2 extra tablespoons of olive oil for the anchovies.

Ingredients

SERVES 4

METRIC (IMPERIAL)	AMERICAN
4 medium-sized waxy potatoes, scrubbed and halved	4 medium-sized
1 medium head of cauliflower, broken into florets	1 medium
2 tablespoons olive oil	2 tablespoons
6 anchovies plus 2 tablespoons oil from the tin	6
2 cloves garlic, crushed	2
juice of 2 lemons	juice of 2
salt and pepper	

Method

1 Steam the potatoes for 15–20 minutes until just cooked.
2 At the same time, steam the cauliflower in a separate pan for 8–12 minutes, until just cooked but still slightly crunchy.
3 Heat the oil in a heavy, wide pan and add the anchovies, their oil and the garlic. Cook for several minutes or until the anchovies have partially dissolved.
4 Add the lemon juice and a little salt and pepper, then add the potatoes, cut into large dice, and the cauliflower florets.
5 Toss well in the sauce and leave to marinate for at least 30 minutes before serving warm or at room temperature.

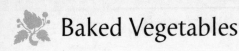 # Baked Vegetables

Wheat/gluten-free 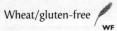 **WF**   Dairy-free **DF**

If you keep a reasonable stock of fresh, tinned or frozen vegetables and some nuts or seeds, you can always create a speedy, tasty, nutritious meal. Use the following selection to give you ideas. This combination will make for a high-fibre meal.

Ingredients

SERVES 4

METRIC (IMPERIAL)	AMERICAN
3 tablespoons olive or sunflower oil	3 tablespoons
1–2 leeks, trimmed and sliced thickly	1–2
4 cloves garlic, peeled and left whole or halved lengthways	4
1 chilli pepper (deseeded and sliced thinly) *or*	1
1 small piece fresh ginger, peeled and cut into small matchsticks (optional)	1 small piece
2 medium-sized potatoes, sweet potatoes or parsnips, peeled/scrubbed and sliced thickly	2 medium-sized
2 handfuls green beans (any kind), trimmed and sliced	2 handfuls
2 courgettes (small zucchini), wiped and sliced thickly	2
2 large handfuls (approx. 100g/4oz) fresh/frozen spinach or Cos lettuce, chopped roughly	2 large handfuls (approx. 4oz)
8 mini tomatoes *or*	8
4 ordinary tomatoes, quartered	4
100g (4oz) smoked/marinated tofu (bean curd), cubed (optional)	4oz
2 tablespoons pumpkin seeds	2 tablespoons
2 teaspoons dried marjoram or oregano (optional)	2 teaspoons

1 x 400g (14oz) tin chickpeas (garbanzos) or butterbeans, drained	1 x 14oz
2 large handfuls fresh parsley or coriander, chopped roughly	2 large handfuls
2 tablespoons roasted, salted cashew nuts	2 tablespoons
sea salt and freshly ground black pepper, wheat-free tamari, Japanese mirin or sea vegetable seasoning	

Method

1 Pour the oil into a large ovenproof dish and add all the ingredients except the pulses, fresh herbs, nuts and seasonings.

2 Cover with foil and bake in a moderate oven (180°C/350°F/Gas Mark 4), stirring periodically, for an hour or until the vegetables are cooked.

3 Add the pulses, herbs and nuts, mix well and return to the oven for 15 minutes.

4 Season to taste and sprinkle generously with fresh herbs before serving from the pan with the cooking juices.

5 If you are in a hurry, cover the dish with microwave film and microwave for 5–8 minutes first to soften the vegetables. Add the pulses and nuts and return to the oven for 20–30 minutes.

Stir-fried Sprouts
with Ginger and Bean Sprouts

Wheat/gluten-free **WF**   Dairy-free **DF**

This high-fibre dish is an unusual way to cook sprouts, taking them right out of their usual soggy Christmas role.

Ingredients   SERVES 4

METRIC (IMPERIAL)	AMERICAN
2 tablespoons sesame or sunflower oil	2 tablespoons
4 large cloves garlic, peeled and sliced very thinly	4 large
40g (1½oz) fresh ginger root, peeled and sliced very finely	1½oz
400g (14oz) Brussels sprouts, trimmed and sliced finely	14oz
75g (3oz) cashew nuts	3oz
200g (7oz) bean sprouts	7oz
tamari (wheat-free soya sauce) and freshly ground black pepper	

Method

1   Heat the oil in a wok and lightly fry the garlic and ginger for 4–5 minutes, making sure they do not burn.
2   Add the Brussels sprouts and cashew nuts and cook quite fast for 2–3 minutes or until the sprouts are just beginning to soften.
3   Add the bean sprouts and cook for a further 2 minutes.
4   Season to taste with tamari and freshly ground black pepper and serve at once.

Beetroot and Chickpea (Garbanzo) Salad

Wheat/gluten-free 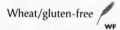 **WF**   Dairy-free **DF**

This high-fibre salad has a wonderful rich colour and flavour.

Ingredients

SERVES 4

METRIC (IMPERIAL)	AMERICAN
2 small raw beetroot, peeled and grated	2 small
400g (14oz) cooked or tinned chickpeas (garbanzos)	14oz
4 large spring onions (scallions), trimmed and chopped	4 large
1 tablespoon tamari or wheat-free soy sauce	1 tablespoon
1 tablespoon vinegar of your choice	1 tablespoon
3 tablespoons olive oil *or*	3 tablespoons
2 tablespoons olive *and*	2 tablespoons
1 tablespoon pumpkin oil	1 tablespoon
freshly ground black pepper	

Method

1 In a covered, microwave-proof dish, mix the grated beetroot thoroughly with the chickpeas (garbanzos) and the spring onions (scallions).

2 Add the tamari, vinegar, oils and pepper and mix again thoroughly.

3 Cover the dish and microwave on full power for 1 minute (warming the chickpeas/garbanzos and beetroot helps them to absorb the dressing), then set aside for 2–3 hours.

4 Mix again thoroughly before serving.

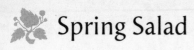

Spring Salad

Wheat/gluten-free 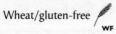 **WF**   Dairy-free **DF**

A delicious combination of cleansing herbs.

Ingredients   SERVES 4

METRIC (IMPERIAL)	AMERICAN
2 bunches watercress	2 bunches
2 large handfuls dandelion leaves	2 large handfuls
6 spring onions (scallions), chopped small	6
1 large bulb fennel, sliced in thin matchsticks	1 large bulb
1 large handful fresh parsley, pulled into small sprigs	1 large handful
leaves from 2 sprigs of fresh thyme	
sea salt and freshly ground black pepper	
juice of 1 lemon	juice of 1
4 tablespoons olive, walnut or hazelnut oil	4 tablespoons
4 nasturtium flowers	4

Method

1 Mix all the herbs and vegetables, except the nasturtium flowers, thoroughly in a bowl.
2 Season with salt and pepper and mix again.
3 Mix the oil and lemon juice and drizzle over the salad.
4 Just before serving, drop on the nasturtium flowers.

Pepper, Pear and Anchovy Salad

Wheat/gluten-free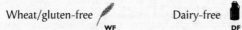
WF

Dairy-free
DF

To make this a vegetarian dish, replace the anchovies with 6–8 pitted black olives, sliced thinly.

Ingredients

SERVES 4

METRIC (IMPERIAL)	AMERICAN
4 tablespoons plain, creamy yoghurt	4 tablespoons
4 anchovy fillets, chopped small	4
freshly ground black pepper	
juice of 1 lemon	juice of 1
1 medium red sweet pepper, deseeded and sliced finely	1 medium
1 medium green sweet pepper, deseeded and sliced finely	1 medium
2 medium pears, peeled and sliced thinly	2 medium
½ head iceberg lettuce	½ head

Method

1 Put the yoghurt in a bowl and add the anchovies (or olives).
2 Mix well, then season to taste with pepper and lemon juice. You should not need any extra salt because of the saltiness of the anchovies.
3 Add the peppers and pears and toss gently until the fruit and vegetables are well coated with the dressing.
4 Serve on a bed of crisp iceberg lettuce.

'An Excellent Salad of Young Vegetables'

Wheat/gluten-free **WF**   Dairy-free **DF**

This Victorian cooked-vegetable salad would be good for anyone who is anxious to keep up their intake of vegetables but finds raw vegetables difficult to digest comfortably.

Ingredients   SERVES 4

METRIC (IMPERIAL)	AMERICAN
300g (10oz) waxy new potatoes, scrubbed, boiled or steamed and sliced	10oz
225g (8oz) young carrots, scrubbed, boiled or steamed and sliced	8oz
4 tablespoons good French dressing	4 tablespoons
approx. 12 cooked artichoke hearts (tinned or frozen), halved	approx. 12
2 tablespoons chopped fresh herbs (e.g. thyme, chives or a mixture of several)	2 tablespoons

Method

1 While still warm, lay the potatoes and carrots out in the bottom of a serving dish and drizzle with half the dressing.
2 Lay the halved artichoke hearts over the potatoes and carrots and drizzle over the rest of the dressing.
3 Just before serving, sprinkle over the fresh herbs.

Winter Cabbage Salad

Wheat/gluten-free 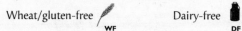 **WF**

Dairy-free   **DF**

The sea vegetables make this a high-fibre salad. It is perfect if you want something really crunchy in the middle of winter.

Ingredients

SERVES 4

METRIC (IMPERIAL)	AMERICAN
75g (3oz) red cabbage, sliced very finely	3oz
50g (2oz) Savoy cabbage, sliced very finely	2oz
50g (2oz) Chinese leaves, sliced very finely	2oz
½ leek, sliced very finely	½
25g (1oz) button mushrooms, sliced finely	1oz
2 large handfuls parsley, chopped	2 large handfuls
50g (2oz) salted, roasted cashew nuts	2oz
1 handful dried Japanese sea vegetables, rehydrated, squeezed out and chopped	1 handful
freshly ground black pepper	
2 tablespoons rice or other vinegar	2 tablespoons
1 tablespoon pumpkin oil	1 tablespoon
4 tablespoons olive oil	4 tablespoons

Method

1   Mix the cabbages, leek, mushrooms, parsley, nuts and sea vegetables.
2   Grind over plenty of black pepper – you should not need any extra salt because the cashew nuts will be salted.
3   Mix the vinegar and oils and use them to dress the salad. You may need to make a little extra if you have sliced the cabbages very finely.

CHAPTER 15

Desserts

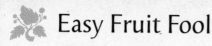

Easy Fruit Fool

Wheat/gluten-free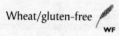

This can be a relatively low-fibre dessert, depending on the fruit you use.

Ingredients

SERVES 4

METRIC (IMPERIAL)	**AMERICAN**
300g (10oz) fresh soft fruit – strawberries, raspberries, peaches, nectarines, apricots etc.	10oz
4 tablespoons plain, live yoghurt	4 tablespoons
½–1 tablespoon maple syrup or dark muscovado sugar	½–1 tablespoon
juice of ½–1 lemon	juice of ½–1

Method

1 Depending on whether you want your fool 'bitty' or smooth, chop the fruit with a knife or purée it in a food processor.
2 Stir the fruit into the yoghurt and flavour it to taste with the maple syrup or muscovado and the lemon juice.
3 Spoon into dishes or glasses and chill before serving.

Hot Plum Dessert

Wheat/gluten-free 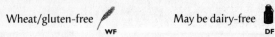 May be dairy-free

A lovely dessert for the soft fruit season. You could also make it with peaches, nectarines or apricots.

Ingredients

SERVES 4

METRIC (IMPERIAL)	AMERICAN
500g (1¼lb) fresh plums	1¼lb
50g (2oz) softened/ready-to-eat prunes	2oz
75g (3oz) dairy-free spread	3oz
50g (2oz) dark muscovado sugar	2oz
75g (3oz) gluten/wheat-free flour *or*	3oz
40g (1½oz) gram (chickpea/garbanzo) flour *and*	1½oz
40g (1½oz) rice flour	1½oz
1 level teaspoon gluten/wheat-free baking powder	1 level teaspoon
2 eggs	2

Method

1 Put half the plums with the prunes in a heavy pan. Cover and cook over a very low heat for 30–45 minutes, stirring regularly, until they have cooked down into a 'marmalade'. Remove the stones.

2 Spread this mixture out in the bottom of an oven-proof pie dish or casserole. Halve the remaining plums and remove their stones. Lay them, cut side up, over the mixture.

3 Heat the oven to 180°C/350°F/Gas Mark 4.

4 Beat the spread with the sugar in an electric mixer until soft and fluffy.

5 Sift the flours with the baking powder.

6 Slowly beat in the eggs, adding a tablespoon of flour with each egg, then fold in the remaining flour.

7 Pour the mixture over the plums and bake for 40 minutes or until a skewer comes out clean.

8 Either serve the pudding from the pie dish or loosen the edges and turn it out onto a serving dish.

9 Serve warm with yoghurt or ice cream.

Blackberry and Apple Crumble

Wheat/gluten-free 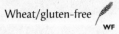 **WF**   May be dairy-free **DF**

This crumble uses only fruits for sweetness, so has no added sugar as such. It also uses polenta and rice flour for the topping so is wheat- and gluten-free – as well as being delicious!

Ingredients

SERVES 4

METRIC (IMPERIAL)	AMERICAN
2 large Bramley cooking (baking) apples *or*	2 large
4 large tart eating apples	4 large
200g (7oz) blackberries	7oz
10 pitted, softened prunes	10
2 tablespoons polenta	2 tablespoons
1 tablespoon rice flour	1 tablespoon
2 tablespoons unsalted cashew nuts	2 tablespoons
1 tablespoon softened dates	1 tablespoon
1 tablespoon dairy-free spread	1 tablespoon

Method

1 Heat the oven to 180°C/350°F/Gas Mark 4.
2 Peel, core and slice the apples and put in a pan with the blackberries, prunes and 4 tablespoons of water. Cover and cook gently for 10 minutes until the fruits are quite soft. Spoon into an ovenproof flan dish.
3 Mix the polenta and rice flour together.
4 Pulverize the cashew nuts with the dates in a food processor and mix into the flours.
5 Rub in the dairy-free spread then distribute the mixture over the top of the fruit.
6 Bake for 30 minutes or until the topping is lightly tanned.
7 Serve alone or with a plain yoghurt.

Chocolate, Orange and Coconut Cream Mousse

Wheat/gluten-free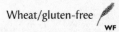
WF

Dairy-free
DF

A rich, yummy and low-fibre dessert.

Ingredients

SERVES 4

METRIC (IMPERIAL)	AMERICAN
150g (5oz) really good, dairy-free, dark chocolate	5oz
3g (½ sachet) gelatin	½ sachet
grated rind and juice of 1 large orange	
3 large eggs, separated	3 large
4 tablespoons coconut cream	4 tablespoons
2 tablespoons brandy	2 tablespoons
chopped pistachio nuts to decorate	

Method

1   Melt the chocolate over hot water or microwave on high for 2–3 minutes.
2   Dissolve the gelatin in the orange juice (you will need to heat the juice).
3   Beat the orange rind, egg yolks, coconut cream and brandy into the chocolate mixture, then add the gelatin melted in the orange juice. Set aside.
4   Whisk the egg whites until they hold their shape in soft peaks, then fold them into the chocolate mixture.
5   Pour into 4 sundae dishes. Cover and refrigerate until the mousse sets. Decorate with the chopped pistachio nuts.

Yoghurt Apricot Cheesecake

Wheat/gluten-free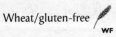

This is a versatile recipe. You can use the apricot mixture without the cake as a mousse, and you can use the sponge as a cake (see page 188).

Ingredients

SERVES 4

METRIC (IMPERIAL)	AMERICAN
2 eggs	2
50g (2oz) caster sugar	2oz
50g (2oz) rice flour	2oz
400g (14oz) fresh, stoned apricots (or dried in the winter)	14oz
1 packet gelatin	1 packet
300g (11oz) set natural yoghurt	11oz

Method

1 Heat the oven to 180°C/350°F/Gas Mark 4.

2 Beat the eggs with the sugar until light and fluffy, then fold in the rice flour.

3 Pour the mixture into a 20cm/8-inch cake tin with a removable bottom and bake for 20 minutes or until the cake is risen and just firm to the touch. Remove from the oven and allow it to cool in the tin.

4 Meanwhile, simmer the stoned apricots very gently in just enough water to cover them. If fresh, they will need only a couple of minutes; if dried, slightly longer. In either case, remove them as soon as they are soft.

5 Carefully remove 8 apricot halves with a slotted spoon and reserve to cover the top of the cheesecake. Drain the rest, reserving the liquid, and purée them in a food processor.

6 Dissolve the gelatin in 3 tablespoons of the cooking liquid.

7 In a bowl, mix the yoghurt thoroughly. Add 2 tablespoons of the apricot purée to the gelatin and then mix it into the yoghurt.

8 Pour this mixture over the cake in the tin and arrange the apricot halves on top.

9 Chill for several hours until the mixture is set, then carefully remove it from the tin and place on a serving dish.

Winter Dried Fruit Compote

Wheat/gluten-free 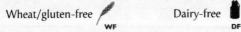 **WF**   Dairy-free **DF**

This compote is excellent warm or cold, for breakfast, lunch or supper, by itself or with yoghurt, fromage frais or ice cream. It has no added sugar and can be high in fibre if you include prunes, figs and apricots; much lower if you stick to sultanas (seedless white raisins), raisins, apples, pears etc. Ideally, the fruits will be pre-softened, but if not you may need to simmer them for 45–60 minutes to make sure they are really soft.

Ingredients

SERVES 4

METRIC (IMPERIAL)	AMERICAN
300g (11oz) dried fruits in any combination – prunes, figs, dates, sultanas (seedless white raisins), cherries, raisins, apples, pears, pineapple etc.	11oz
600ml (1 pint) water	2½ cups
½ lemon, sliced	½
1 stick vanilla or cinnamon	1 stick

Method

1   Put all the ingredients together in a pan, cover and bring very slowly to the boil.
2   Simmer for 30 minutes.
3   Strain the fruit, reserving the cooking liquid, and put it in a serving bowl.
4   Return the juices to the heat, with the lemon and cinnamon or vanilla stick, and continue to simmer briskly for 5–10 minutes until slightly reduced.
5   Pour over the fruit and allow to cool.
6   Serve warm, at room temperature or chilled, as you prefer.

Cranberry Rice Pudding with Rice Milk

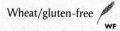 Wheat/gluten-free

WF

May be dairy-free

DF

For those used to low-sugar dishes, this will be delicious. Those used to sweeter puddings may need to add a tablespoon of maple syrup or muscovado sugar. You can also substitute sultanas (seedless white raisins) for the cranberries to make a more conventional – and slightly sweeter – pudding. Made with sultanas (seedless white raisins), the pudding is very low-fibre; with cranberries, slightly higher.

Ingredients

SERVES 4

METRIC (IMPERIAL)	AMERICAN
50g (2oz) short-grain white rice	2oz
25g (1oz) cranberries or sultanas (seedless white raisins)	1oz
300ml (10fl oz) vanilla-flavoured rice milk *or*	1¼ cups
300ml (10fl oz) plain rice milk heated just to boiling point with a vanilla pod, *or*	1¼ cups
300ml (10fl oz) plain rice milk with 1 teaspoon good quality vanilla essence	1¼ cups

Method

1 Heat the oven to 170°C/325°F/Gas Mark 3 – unless you have an Aga, in which case the bottom oven is ideal.

2 Put the rice, cranberries and milk (discarding the vanilla pod if used) into an oven-proof dish and mix around.

3 Cook uncovered, very slowly, for 2½–3 hours, stirring occasionally.

4 Serve warm or cold, alone or with yoghurt or fromage frais.

Wheat-free Pancakes

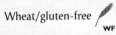

Wheat/gluten-free
WF

May be dairy-free
DF

Neither sweet nor savoury, these pancakes can be used for a dessert or a main-course dish. They freeze well, as long as they are interleaved with clingfilm or greaseproof (wax) paper so you can peel off as many as you need. Defrost them briefly in a microwave. You can use any of the fillings below or make up your own.

Ingredients

SERVES 4

METRIC (IMPERIAL)	AMERICAN
75g (4oz) gram (chickpea/garbanzo) flour	4oz
25g (1oz) white rice flour	1oz
pinch salt	pinch
200ml (7fl oz) water	⁷/₈ cup
1 egg, beaten	1
1 tablespoon sunflower oil	1 tablespoon

Filling

juice of 2 lemons	juice of 2
50g (2oz) caster sugar *or*	2oz
4 tablespoons good fruit jam (jelly)	4 tablespoons
4 tablespoons plain yoghurt or fromage frais *or*	4 tablespoons
4 tablespoons puréed apple	4 tablespoons
4 tablespoons broken walnuts	4 tablespoons

Method

1 Whizz the flours, salt, water and egg in a food processor then allow to stand for 10–15 minutes.
2 Heat a pancake pan with a tiny dribble of oil. Pour one small ladleful of the mixture into the pan and cook quickly on both sides. The pancakes should be quite thick and you should get at least 8 out of the mixture.
3 If they are to be eaten at once, serve them from the pan with sugar and lemon juice or filling of your choice.
4 If they are to be used later, stack them with a piece of clingfilm or greaseproof (wax) paper between each pancake.

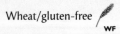

Baked Fruit Flan

Wheat/gluten-free
WF

This combination of fruit is available more or less year-round, but you could change it for more seasonal fruits if you wished. This recipe is moderately high in fibre.

Ingredients

SERVES 4

METRIC (IMPERIAL)	AMERICAN
1 tablespoon apple and pear concentrate or spread	1 tablespoon
1 x 20cm (8-inch) precooked pastry case (see recipe for gluten/wheat-free pastry, page 175)	1 x 8-inch
1 Bramley cooking (baking) apple *or*	1
2 medium tart eating apples	2 medium
1 large orange	1 large
2 kiwi fruit	2
125g (5oz) fromage frais	5oz
25g (1oz) browned, flaked almonds	1oz

Method

1 Heat the oven to 180°C/350°F/Gas Mark 4.
2 Spread the pear and apple concentrate over the bottom of the pastry case.
3 Peel, core and slice the apple and lay it over the concentrate.
4 Peel and thinly slice the orange and lay it over the apple, then do the same with the kiwi fruit.
5 Cover with foil and bake for 20 minutes. Remove from the oven and allow to cool slightly.
6 Spread the fromage frais over the fruit and sprinkle over the flaked almonds.
7 Serve warm or at room temperature.

Banana and Date Chocolate Ice Cream

Wheat/gluten-free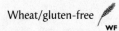
WF

May be dairy-free
DF

You will need an ice-cream maker for this recipe as it is not only sugar-free but almost fat-free and fibre-free. If you want to make it richer and creamier, you could substitute coconut cream or soya cream, or goat's or cow's milk cream for the soya, oat or rice milk.

Ingredients

SERVES 4

METRIC (IMPERIAL)	AMERICAN
50g (2oz) dried dates, softened in boiling water if very hard, and chopped roughly	2oz
2 medium bananas	2 medium
300ml (10fl oz) unsweetened soya milk, unsweetened oat milk or rice milk	1¼ cups
40g (1½oz) cocoa powder	1½oz

Method

1. Mash the dates with the bananas in a food processor.
2. Heat the milk and pour it over the cocoa powder, mixing gently to make a smooth paste. Add this to the banana and dates and whizz very thoroughly. Cool.
3. Pour the mixture into an ice-cream maker and churn freeze.
4. If you are not eating it immediately, remove the ice cream from the freezer and soften for 30 minutes in a fridge before serving.

Passion Fruit Yoghurt Ice Cream

Wheat/gluten-free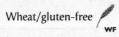
WF

Ingredients

SERVES 4

METRIC (IMPERIAL)	**AMERICAN**
200g (7oz) Greek-style yoghurt	7oz
6 passion fruit	6
juice of 1–2 lemons	juice of 1–2
50g (2oz) pale muscovado sugar	2oz

Method

1 Beat the yoghurt in a bowl with a wooden spoon or whisk until quite smooth.
2 Halve the passion fruit and scoop the flesh into the yoghurt.
3 Add the lemon juice and sugar to taste, remembering that freezing dulls the flavour so the mixture should be over- rather than under-flavoured before freezing.
4 Turn the mixture into an ice-cream maker and churn freeze.
5 If the ice cream is not to be eaten immediately, remove from the freezer and store in the fridge for 20–30 minutes before serving to allow the mixture to soften slightly.

CHAPTER 16

Baking

Rice Flour and Banana Bread

Wheat/gluten-free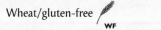
WF

Dairy-free
DF

This low-fibre loaf has more of the texture of a cake than of bread but tastes 'bready'.

Ingredients

MAKES 1 SMALL LOAF

METRIC (IMPERIAL)	**AMERICAN**
2 medium bananas	2 medium
150g (5oz) rice flour	5oz
50g (2oz) dairy-free spread	2oz
2 heaped teaspoons wheat/gluten-free baking powder	2 heaped teaspoons
1 egg	1
100ml (3½fl oz) rice, soya or coconut milk	½ cup

Method

1 Heat the oven to 180°C/350°F/Gas Mark 4.
2 Purée the bananas in a food processor along with all the other ingredients.
3 Line the bottom of a small loaf tin with greaseproof (wax) paper and oil its sides.
4 Spoon the mixture into the tin and bake for 35 minutes or until a skewer comes out clean.
5 Remove from the oven and allow to cool slightly. Knock out of the tin and place on a rack to cool, covered with a tea towel.

Gluten- and Wheat-free
Shortcrust Pastry

Wheat/gluten-free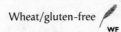
WF

Dairy-free
DF

Ingredients

MAKES 1 X 20CM (8-INCH) FLAN CASE

METRIC (IMPERIAL)	AMERICAN
75g (3oz) dairy-free spread	3oz
75g (3oz) rice flour	3oz
75g (3oz) sifted gram (chickpea/garbanzo) flour	3oz
3 tablespoons water	3 tablespoons

Method

1 Heat the oven to 180°C/350°F/Gas Mark 4.
2 Rub the spread into the flours then add enough water to make a soft dough.
3 Roll out the pastry carefully and use it to line a round or oval flan dish with a removable base. Cover with foil or greaseproof (wax) paper and weight with beans. Bake the pastry for 10 minutes then remove the foil and return to the oven for another 10 minutes to crisp the pastry.

Oaten 'Soda' Bread

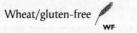 Wheat/gluten-free Dairy-free

The oats give this bread a very good flavour and texture. If you need to avoid oats, you can substitute sifted gram (chickpea/garbanzo) flour. You will need to cook the bread for an extra 5 minutes and it will have a rather more dense, but still very acceptable, texture.

Ingredients

METRIC (IMPERIAL)	AMERICAN
250g (9oz) porridge oats, processed until very fine	9oz
200g (7oz) brown rice flour	7oz
2 heaped teaspoons cream of tartar	2 heaped teaspoons
1 heaped teaspoon bicarbonate of soda (baking soda)	1 heaped teaspoon
1 heaped teaspoon soya flour	1 heaped teaspoon
1 heaped teaspoon xanthan gum	1 heaped teaspoon
1 level teaspoon sugar	1 level teaspoon
1 level teaspoon salt	1 level teaspoon
25g (1oz) dairy-free spread	1oz
1 large egg	1 large
200ml (7fl oz) rice, oat or soya milk	⅞ cup

Method

1 Heat the oven to 190°C/375°F/Gas Mark 5.
2 Mix together all the dry ingredients thoroughly in a large mixing bowl, then rub in the spread.
3 Mix in the egg, followed by the milk, making sure there are no lumps.
4 Grease a baking tray.
5 Form the bread into a round loaf and cut a cross in the centre.
6 Bake for 40 minutes or until the bread is risen and a skewer comes out clean.
7 Remove from the oven onto a wire rack and cover with a tea towel. Make sure the bread is quite cold before slicing.

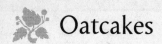# Oatcakes

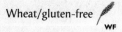
Wheat/gluten-free **WF**   Dairy-free **DF**

Great with any kind of spread or nut butter, on their own or with salad.

Ingredients

MAKES AROUND 10

METRIC (IMPERIAL)	AMERICAN
100g (4oz) rolled oats, pulverized in a processor	4oz
50g (2oz) rice flour	2oz
½ teaspoon gluten/wheat-free baking powder	½ teaspoon
¼ teaspoon salt	¼ teaspoon
1 tablespoon dairy-free spread	1 tablespoon

Method

1   Heat the oven to 180°C/350°F/Gas Mark 4.
2   Mix the oats with the rice flour, baking powder and salt and rub in the spread.
3   Add enough cold water to mix to a soft dough then roll out. You can make it as thick or thin as you want but no thinner than 5mm (¼ inch).
4   Transfer the oatcakes to a baking tray and bake for 10–15 minutes, depending on how thick you made them. Cool on a rack before eating.

Ginger Biscuits

Wheat/gluten-free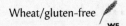
WF

Dairy-free
DF

As with all biscuits free of wheat flour, these are pretty crumbly so need to be treated with care. But they are delicious so it is worth the effort!

Ingredients

MAKES AROUND 12

METRIC (IMPERIAL)	AMERICAN
40g (1½oz) light muscovado sugar	1½oz
60g (2oz) rice flour	2oz
40g (1½oz) gram (chickpea/garbanzo) flour	1½oz
2 teaspoons ground ginger	2 teaspoons
pinch salt	pinch
75g (3oz) dairy-free spread	3oz

Method

1   Heat the oven to 170°C/325°F/Gas Mark 3.

2   Mix the sugar, flours, ginger and salt in a bowl then rub in the spread – you can use a pastry mixer for this.

3   Press the mixture out into a baking tin about 10cm (½-inch) thick and bake for 10 minutes.

4   Remove from the oven and cut the mixture into biscuit shapes, then return to the oven for a further 5 minutes or until the biscuits are golden.

5   Cool and remove with care so they do not crumble.

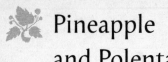

Pineapple
and Polenta Christmas Cake

Wheat/gluten-free 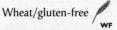 **WF**　　　　Dairy-free　**DF**

*This delicious, fresh-tasting, rich fruit cake has no refined sugar and is
quite high in fibre. If the dates or pears are very hard or dry, soften for
10 minutes in boiling water.*

Ingredients

Metric (Imperial)	American
200g (7oz) dairy-free spread	7oz
100g (4oz) each soft dried dates and pears, puréed	4oz
3 eggs	3
100g (4oz) coarse polenta	4oz
100g (4oz) white rice or potato flour	4oz
2 heaped teaspoons wheat/gluten-free baking powder	2 heaped teaspoons
50g (2oz) fresh or tinned pineapple	2oz
50g (2oz) sultanas (seedless white raisins)	2oz
50g (2oz) cherries	2oz
2 tablespoons elderflower cordial	2 tablespoons

Method

1   Heat the oven to 180°C/350°F/Gas Mark 4.

2   Beat the spread with the puréed dates and pears until smooth and creamy.

3   Mix in the eggs then mix/fold in the polenta sieved with the rice or potato flour and the baking powder.

4   Cut the pineapple into small pieces and stir it into the mixture along with the sultanas (seedless white raisins), cherries and elderflower cordial.

5   Spoon into a well-oiled 20cm (8-inch) baking tin and bake for 30 minutes or until the cake is firm to the touch and a skewer comes out clean.

6   Cool on a rack.

Apple and Cinnamon Cake

Wheat/gluten-free 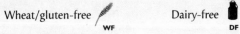 WF   Dairy-free DF

This delicious, moist, spicy, light fruit cake has no added sugar and relatively little fibre.

Ingredients

METRIC (IMPERIAL)	AMERICAN
100g (4oz) dairy-free spread	4oz
200g (7oz) dried dates, finely chopped	7oz
225g (8oz) tart eating apples, cored, peeled and grated	8oz
2 heaped teaspoons ground cinnamon	2 heaped teaspoons
1 level teaspoon ground mixed spice	1 level teaspoon
pinch salt	pinch
75g (3oz) raisins	3oz
2 medium eggs	2 medium
140g (5oz) rice flour	5oz
140g (5oz) gram (chickpea/garbanzo) flour	5oz
2 heaped teaspoons gluten/wheat-free baking powder	2 heaped teaspoons
180ml (6fl oz) rice, soya or oat milk	¾ cup

Method

1 Preheat the oven to 180°C/350°F/Gas Mark 4 and grease and line a 20cm (8-inch) square tin.

2 Put the spread, dates, apples, cinnamon, mixed spice and salt into a processor and blend thoroughly.

3 Fold in the raisins and eggs, alternately with the flour, baking powder and milk.

4 When all ingredients are amalgamated, transfer the mixture to the tin.

5 Bake for 30–40 minutes until dark golden and firm to the touch. Test with a skewer.

6 Remove from the oven and leave to cool in the tin for 10–15 minutes before turning onto a wire rack to cool completely.

Chocolate and Prune Cake

Wheat/gluten-free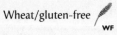
WF

Dairy-free
DF

This delicious chocolate cake can be converted into a rather luscious dessert. Simply split it horizontally, fill with a jam (jelly) of your choice, then top with fromage frais and grated chocolate. If you wish to reduce the fibre content, replace the prunes and banana with 140g (5oz) dark muscovado sugar.

Ingredients

METRIC (IMPERIAL)	AMERICAN
140g (5oz) ready-to-eat prunes	5oz
1 large banana	1 large
140g (5oz) dairy-free spread	5oz
250g (9oz) dairy-free chocolate	9oz
3 medium eggs	3 medium
75g (3oz) sifted gram (chickpea/garbanzo) flour	3oz
75g (3oz) rice flour	3oz
1 heaped teaspoon gluten/wheat-free baking powder	1 heaped teaspoon
1–2 tablespoons whatever milk you can have	1–2 tablespoons

Method

1 Heat the oven to 180°C/350°F/Gas Mark 4.
2 Grease and line a 20cm (8-inch) cake tin.
3 Chop the prunes finely in a food processor, then add the banana.
4 Beat the spread in a food mixer, then add the prune and banana mixture. Beat thoroughly.
5 Melt the chocolate over hot water or in a microwave, then beat it into the mixture.
6 Beat in the eggs, one at a time, each accompanied by a spoonful of flour.
7 Fold in the rest of the flour and baking powder, adding a little milk if needed, and turn into the cake tin.
8 Bake for 30 minutes or until a skewer comes out clean.

Chocolate (or Cinnamon) Muffins

Wheat/gluten-free
WF

Dairy-free
DF

If you want to convert these into cinnamon muffins, substitute a heaped teaspoon of cinnamon for the heaped tablespoon of cocoa powder (unsweetened cocoa).

Ingredients

MAKES 6 MUFFINS

METRIC (IMPERIAL)	AMERICAN
100g (4oz) rolled oats, pulverized in a food processor	4oz
25g (2oz) rice flour	2oz
1 large, heaped tablespoon pure cocoa powder (unsweetened cocoa)	1 large, heaped tablespoon
1 heaped teaspoon gluten/wheat-free baking powder	1 heaped teaspoon
100g (4oz) soft dried dates, chopped very small in a food processor	4oz
75g (3oz) dairy-free spread	3oz
1 egg	1
120ml (4fl oz) soya, oat, rice or coconut milk	½ cup
50g (2oz) broken cashew nuts	2oz

Method

1 Heat the oven to 180°C/350°F/Gas Mark 4 and oil some large mince pie/muffin tins or large paper cake cases.

2 Put the pulverized oats, rice flour, cocoa (or cinnamon), baking powder, dates and dairy-free spread into a food processor and whizz until puréed.

3 Add the egg and milk and whizz again.

4 Remove the blade from the processor and stir in the nuts.

5 Spoon the mixture into the mince pie/muffin tins or cake cases and bake for 20 minutes or until a skewer comes out clean.

6 Cool on a rack before eating.

Light Sponge or Angel Cake

Wheat/gluten-free **WF**   Dairy-free **DF**

This is excellent on its own sprinkled with a little icing (powdered) sugar and layered with jam (jelly), but it also makes a first-class base for a wide range of desserts. It is very low in fibre.

Ingredients

Metric (Imperial)	American
6 medium eggs	6 medium
150g (5oz) caster sugar	5oz
150g (5oz) rice flour	5oz

Method

1 Heat the oven to 170°C/325°F/Gas Mark 3.

2 Line a loose-bottomed 20cm (8-inch) cake tin with lightly floured greaseproof (wax) paper.

3 Whisk the eggs and sugar together with an electric whisk until light and fluffy (4–5 minutes).

4 Sift the flour into the bowl and fold carefully into the egg mixture, making sure you leave no lumps of flour.

5 Pour the mixture into the tin and bake for 20–30 minutes or until the cake is firm to the touch.

6 Remove from the oven and, carefully, from the tin. Peel off the greaseproof (wax) paper and allow to cool on a rack, then fill with jam (jelly) and sprinkle with icing (powdered) sugar as for a normal sponge cake.

7 If you are to use the cake in another recipe (such as for a trifle or tiramisu), it will freeze well.

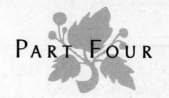

PART FOUR

Taking it Further

CHAPTER 17

Helpful nutritional supplements

This chapter looks at nutritional supplements that may be helpful to I.B.S. sufferers.

Probiotics

Supplements containing probiotic bacteria – and substances that promote their growth – are among the most widely used. Probiotic bacteria encourage 'friendly' microbes, such as Lactobacilli and Bifidobacteria, to colonize the bowel. This creates a healthy intestinal environment, which discourages infection by potentially harmful, disease-causing bacteria.

Prebiotics describes the use of food substances, such as fructo-oligosaccharides (FOS) and oatmeal, that promote the growth of probiotic bacteria. FOS cannot be digested or absorbed from the human bowel, but act as a fermentable food source for probiotic bacteria in the gut. In contrast, harmful bacteria, such as E. coli and Clostridium, cannot use FOS as a source of energy. Dietary sources of FOS include garlic, onions, barley, wheat, bananas, honey and tomatoes.

The intestines of an average, healthy adult contain around 11 trillion bacteria, weighing up to 1.5 kilograms (3½ pounds). Ideally, at least 70 per cent of these should be healthy probiotic bacteria, and only 30 per cent other bowel bacteria, such as E. coli. In practice, however, the balance is usually the other way round.

Studies have found, for example, that people with I.B.S. consistently have significantly lower amounts of Lactobacilli and Bifidobacteria in their bowels compared with non-I.B.S. sufferers. This may lead to a bacterial imbalance known as dysbiosis, which has been linked with diarrhoea, I.B.S., inflammatory bowel disease and other gastrointestinal problems.

Probiotic bacteria help to reduce the overgrowth of harmful yeast and bacteria in the intestines in a number of different ways. They produce lactic acid, acetic acid and hydrogen peroxide that increase the acidity of the intestines, discouraging less acid-tolerant, harmful bacteria. They have also been shown to secrete natural antibiotics (bacteriocins such as acidophiline and bulgarican) and to stimulate production of interferon, a natural anti-viral agent which helps to protect against viral intestinal infections. They also compete with harmful bacteria for available nutrients, as well as for attachment sites on intestinal cell walls. If these attachment sites are already occupied by friendly bacteria, those that are potentially harmful cannot easily gain a foothold in the intestines and are more likely to be flushed out. These actions are together highly effective, and the presence of friendly, probiotic bacteria improves intestinal health, promotes good digestion, boosts immunity and increases resistance to infection – including traveller's gastroenteritis.

Over 50 trials, involving more than 6000 volunteers in total, have found that probiotic supplements can help treat symptoms associated with a variety of intestinal and other disorders as well as reducing the side-effects brought on by taking antibiotics (such as diarrhoea). They can also reduce wind, bloating and pain.

In one study, 100 patients with I.B.S. were divided into four groups. Twenty patients were given supplements containing active Lactobacilli (a strain known as *L. plantarum 299v*). A further 20 received inactivated bacteria, while the remainder received conventional drug therapy with either mebeverine or trimebutin. In the last group, 22 patients did not improve with drug therapy alone and went on to receive the drug plus probiotic supplements. Results showed a 75 per cent improvement in symptoms among those taking the Lactobacilli, compared with 23 per cent and 30 per cent in those taking the drugs trimebutin and mebeverine. When Lactobacilli were taken in addition to mebeverine, improvements increased to 90 per cent (66 per cent for trimebutin plus Lactobacilli). In contrast, no improvement occurred in those taking an inactivated placebo solution of Lactobacilli. The researchers concluded that enrichment of the colon flora with *L. plantarum* can improve the results of classic drug treatment for I.B.S.

In another study, 60 patients with I.B.S. were divided randomly into two groups, one of which received a fruit-based solution of *L. plantarum* daily for four weeks, while the other received a similar solution – comparable in colour, texture and taste – that contained no bacteria. Flatulence was rapidly and significantly decreased in those drinking the active solution compared with the control group.

A recent study looked at pregnant women with a family history of allergic (atopic) diseases, such as eczema, asthma and rhinitis. During their pregnancy, they were given probiotic supplements of Lactobacillus GG. After delivery, the mothers had the option of giving them to their infants for six months. The frequency of atopic eczema was found to be half that in the babies who had taken active probiotics than in those receiving a placebo. This suggests that bowel bacteria produce a unique effect on the immune system, although this is currently poorly understood. As the immune system is implicated in the development of some forms of food intolerance, taking probiotic supplements may even have a protective action against them.

Probiotic supplements are also thought to help:

* Improve constipation
* Inhibit growth of *Helicobacter pylori,* a bacterium linked with gastritis, gastric ulcers and stomach cancer
* Prevent and treat bowel and vaginal yeast infections caused by *Candida albicans*
* Reduce the formation of cancer-causing substances in the gut by inhibiting the enzymes necessary to produce them
* Lower the risk of breast cancer
* Reduce absorption of ammonia from the intestines in patients with liver disease
* Boost the function of immune cells
* Boost production of protective antibodies
* Counter the development of allergies

* Aid digestion and reduce symptoms of lactose intolerance in susceptible individuals
* Improve symptoms of I.B.S.

Who is likely to be deficient in probiotic bacteria?
Anyone who:

* Has recently taken a course of antibiotics
* Eats a nutrient-poor diet
* Suffers from inflammatory or infective intestinal problems, such as inflammatory bowel disease, chronic diarrhoea, diverticulitis
* Has had a recent course of radiotherapy or chemotherapy
* Is suffering from a serious illness
* Has an immune disorder such as AIDS

Dietary sources of probiotic bacteria include live bio yoghurts and fermented milk drinks. Supplements supply a guaranteed potency of bacteria in capsule, powder, liquid or tablet form. Foods or supplements containing probiotics should normally be kept refrigerated as probiotic bacteria are fragile. A bio yoghurt that has been standing around in the supermarket or in your fridge for a week or more will contain fewer live bacteria than freshly-made cultures.

Ideally, there should be at least one million live Bifidobacterium and/or one million live Acidophilus bacteria per gram of yoghurt for it to achieve its potential health benefits. Levels of live probiotic bacteria in bio yoghurts vary widely, however, from a few hundred thousand to more than 300 million live bacteria per gram. For this reason, it is best to take a probiotic supplement when, for example, aiming to reduce the risk of traveller's diarrhoea abroad.

Dose
When choosing a probiotic supplement, select one that supplies at least 1–2 billion colony-forming units (CFU) of acidophilus per dose. Supplements that are enteric coated – which improves survival of probiotic bacteria as they pass through the acidic stomach – can

contain less (e.g. 10 million freeze-dried probiotic bacteria) and still achieve the same effects.

Probiotic supplements that have been clinically proven to contain bacteria which can reach the bowel, survive there and improve gastrointestinal symptoms, include:

- Yakult (milk-based drink)
- Culturelle (a capsule containing dried probiotic bacteria)
- ProViva (a fruit-based non-dairy drink)
- Multibionta (a tablet combining probiotics with vitamins and minerals)

There are no known problems associated with continuous treatment, even at high dosage.

Aloe vera

Aloe vera is a popular herbal supplement taken to relieve symptoms of I.B.S. There are many species, of which *Aloe barbadensis* is reputed to have the most useful medicinal properties.

Aloe gel is squeezed from the succulent leaves, which can grow to over 60 centimetres (2 feet) long. This contains a unique mix of vitamins, amino acids, enzymes and minerals that have been valued for their healing properties for over 6000 years.

Aloe vera gel contains soapy substances (saponins) that help to cleanse the bowel, and pulpy microfibres (lignins), whose fibre content helps to absorb fluid and toxins from the bowel and bulk up the motions. It has three main healing effects, containing substances that:

- Are anti-inflammatory (anthraquinones and natural plant steroids)
- Hasten wound healing (fibroblast growth factor)
- Are powerful antioxidants (vitamins C, E, betacarotene)
- Are antiseptic (saponins and anthraquinones) and help kill some bacteria, viruses and fungi

Aloe vera juice can be made from fresh liquid extract (gel) or from powdered aloe. The fresh gel has to be stabilized within hours of harvesting to prevent oxidation, which destroys its effectiveness. When selecting a product, aim for one made from 100 per cent pure aloe vera. Its strength needs to be at least 40 per cent by volume to be effective, and ideally approaching 95 per cent. Also, choose one made from aloe liquid rather than powder. You may find it more palatable to choose a product containing a little natural fruit juice (such as grape or apple), although some sufferers find that fruit juice makes their symptoms worse.

Some aloe vera products contain the bitter aloe 'latex' extracted from the inner yellow leaves of the plant. This has a powerful cathartic effect, and taking too much will produce a brisk laxative response due to the presence of chemicals known as anthraquinones (e.g. aloin, which has a bitter taste). These chemicals stimulate contraction of the smooth-muscle fibres lining the bowel and usually work within eight to twelve hours. This can be a desirable effect, of course, if you are experiencing constipation. Many products claim to be aloin- and emodin-free, but independent laboratory tests on leading brands in the US found high levels of aloin in juice which purported to be aloin-free. It is therefore worth selecting a product carrying the IASC (International Aloe Science Council) certified seal, which shows it has been produced according to recommended guidelines.

Dose

If taking the aloe latex for its laxative effect, start with a small dose of gel (e.g. one teaspoon) and work up to around 1–2 tablespoons per day to find the dose that suits you best.

Aloe vera juice may be taken more liberally (e.g. 50–100 ml three times daily). Some women using aloe vera notice that it increases their menstrual flow.

Taking aloe vera by mouth should be avoided in pregnancy as the anthraquinones it may contain can stimulate uterine contractions, which could result in miscarriage. It should also be avoided when breastfeeding as it can trigger stomach cramps and diarrhoea in infants.

Artichoke *(Cynara scolymus)*

Globe artichoke leaves contain several unique substances, such as cynarin, cynaropicrin and cynaroside, that can increase bile secretion and significantly improve digestive symptoms such as bloating, flatulence, nausea and abdominal pain due to intestinal spasm.

Bile is a yellow-green fluid made in the liver and stored in the gall bladder until needed. When food leaves the stomach and enters the first section of the small intestines (duodenum), this triggers a reflex contraction of the gall bladder, which squirts bile into the duodenum where it mixes with food. Bile contains salts and acids that break down fat globules into smaller particles (emulsification) so they can be absorbed and processed more easily. Studies have shown that taking 320 mg of artichoke extracts can increase bile secretion by over 127 per cent after 30 minutes, 151 per cent after 60 minutes, and 94 per cent after 90 minutes.

In one study of 279 people with dyspeptic syndrome who also had symptoms compatible with I.B.S., such as bloating, spasm and impaired gastrointestinal function, 96 per cent found that standardized cynara artichoke supplements were as effective, if not better, than previous treatments they had taken. Overall, I.B.S. symptoms were reduced by 71 per cent within an average of 10 days, although a third noticed an effect within one week. During the six-week study, only three people developed adverse effects that were thought to be associated with artichoke leaf extracts. These were hunger in one person and temporary increase in flatulence in two.

Another study involving over 550 people found that taking artichoke extracts for six weeks could reduce nausea by 82 per cent, vomiting by 88 per cent, bloating by 66 per cent, abdominal pain by 76 per cent, constipation by 71 per cent, fat intolerance by 59 per cent, and swelling of lower legs by 46 per cent.

Dose

One to six 320 mg capsules of artichoke extracts are taken daily, with food. If you have gallstones, consult your doctor before taking this supplement. It should not be taken if you have any obstruction of your bile ducts. No serious adverse reactions to this supplement have been reported.

Chamomile *(Matricaria chamomilla or M. recutita)*

German chamomile has anti-inflammatory, antacid, anti-parasitic, antispasmodic and sedative actions. It helps to relieve intestinal spasm associated with wind, colic and I.B.S., and can also relieve menstrual cramps. It has a mild sedative action, helping to reduce anxiety and stress and to promote sleep.

Dose

Drink one to three cups of chamomile tea daily.

Dandelion *(Taraxacum officinalis)*

Dandelion is a well-known perennial weed whose root (usually obtained from two-year old plants) is widely used for liver and digestive problems. Dandelion root works on the liver, increasing detoxification functions and stimulating the flow of bile so more toxins are eliminated through the bowel. It also has a gentle laxative action that helps to improve constipation. Dandelion leaf also has a diuretic action, helping to increase the elimination of water-soluble toxins from the body and improving feelings of bloating.

Dose

Take 500 mg extracts, twice a day. Side-effects are uncommon, but large doses can cause nausea and diarrhoea. Do not use dandelion if you have active gallstones or obstructive jaundice.

Flaxseed *(Linum usitatissimum)*

Flaxseed (also known as linseed) is the richest known plant source of an omega-3 essential fatty acid, alpha-linolenic acid, which is similar to the essential fatty acids (EFAs) found in fish oil, but less potent. This has an anti-inflammatory, soothing effect on the bowel. Flaxseed oils also contain a beneficial omega-6 essential fatty acid, linolenic acid. Flaxseed is a good fibre source and is useful for improving constipation, diverticular disease and I.B.S.

Take 1 to 2 tablespoons of flaxseeds with water, twice a day. This supplement is best taken with food to enhance absorption.

Garlic *(Allium sativum)*

Garlic has a number of medicinal uses and is antioxidant, antiseptic, antibacterial and antiviral. Garlic is often used to treat diarrhoea, wind and indigestion, although if raw cloves are eaten excessively, they can actually produce flatulence. As a source of fructo-oligosaccharides, garlic promotes a healthy intestinal balance. Garlic has the additional benefits of lowering high blood pressure, beneficially changing blood fat ratios to reduce the risk of heart disease, and improving blood flow to the extremities and brain.

Dose

Take 600 mg to 900 mg daily. You may opt for coated garlic powder tablets, as these reduce the odour on your breath and protect the active ingredients from breaking down in the stomach.

Ginger *(Zingiber officinale)*

Ginger is one of the oldest known medicinal spices and is used to improve a number of intestinal symptoms such as nausea, indigestion, flatulence and diarrhoea. Its rhizome contains a variety of unique chemicals such as gingerol, zingerone and essential oils.

Dose

Powdered ginger root standardized for 0.4 per cent volatile oils: 250 mg two to four times daily. Fresh powdered ginger: 1–2 grams every four hours as necessary. There is no evidence of any side-effects but do not exceed recommended doses during pregnancy.

Goldenseal *(Hydrastis canadensis)*

The herb goldenseal contains many unique substances, including alkaloids such as hydrastine and canadine. It has a natural antibacterial and antiviral action, and boosts immunity by activating the body's scavenger cells, known as macrophages. Goldenseal is widely used to overcome infections and to improve nausea and vomiting. It helps to normalize muscular action in the bowel, and is therefore advised by some practitioners to treat either constipation or diarrhoea in I.B.S.

Dose

Take a 125 mg extract two to four times daily (standardized to at least 8 per cent alkaloids or 5 per cent hydrastine). Goldenseal is usually taken only for up to two weeks at a time. Do not use during pregnancy or while breastfeeding, or if you have high blood pressure or glaucoma. Very high doses may cause mouth dryness.

Kava kava *(Piper methysticum)*

The root of kava kava contains a variety of unique pyrones (e.g. kavain), kavalactones and flavokavins that can reduce anxiety, panic attacks and insomnia due to stress. Kava is mildly sedative, promotes feelings of relaxation and calm, relieves muscle tension and is helpful for mild to moderate pain, especially where due to muscle spasm as in I.B.S.

The anxiety-reducing effects may be noticed with just a single dose, taken as required, while the other effects are usually noticeable within a week of starting treatment and continue to improve over the next month. A trial involving 101 people with generalized anxiety, tension, agoraphobia, social phobia, insomnia and panic attacks found that kava produced an improvement in most participants within two months. By three months, the average anxiety score had dropped from 30.7 to 13.4, and down to 9.9 by six months. Other studies suggest it is as effective as some prescription drugs in treating mild to moderate anxiety, and that it can significantly improve anxiety, depression and insomnia in women with menopausal symptoms.

DOSE

Take 120 mg kava pyrones daily. Products standardized to 30 per cent kavalactones: 250 mg three times a day. Products standardized to 70 per cent kavalactones: 100 mg three times a day. Kava may be taken on an as-needed basis, which for some people may be every day. For example, a single 120 mg kava tablet can be used to produce an immediate calming effect before a stressful event, or to help relieve insomnia associated with anxiety. For someone with persistent anxiety, however, kava needs to be taken daily for 10 to 14 days to produce its full anxiety-reducing action.

Some kava teas may provide over 200 mg kavalactones per cup, so do not over-indulge. Do not combine kava with alcohol (may cause nausea, stomach upsets or sedation), other tranquillizers or illegal drugs. Kava should not be taken during pregnancy or when breast-feeding. Kava should not be taken by people with Parkinson's disease as it may affect dopamine levels and produce abnormal movements.

Excessive use of kava at greater than recommended doses can cause dizziness, grogginess, muscle weakness and visual disturbances. High doses (equivalent to 400mg or more of purified kava lactones per day) may result in a temporary yellow discolouration of the skin or a reversible scaly skin rash known as kani. Excess can also affect liver function and is not recommended.

Lemon balm *(Melissa officinalis)*

Lemon balm contains a variety of aromatic essential oils and is used for its soothing, calming properties. It was also known as the 'Scholar's Herb' as it was traditionally taken by students suffering from the stress of impending exams. It has sedative, anti-spasmodic and antibacterial actions and is widely used to ease a number of stress-related symptoms including digestive problems, nausea, flatulence, depression, tenseness, restlessness, irritability, anxiety, headaches and insomnia.

When combined with valerian, the two herbs work in synergy to reduce symptoms of tension, stress and mild depression. They also have a gentle lowering effect on the raised blood pressure that often accompanies stress.

Dose

Take 650 mg, three times a day. Do not take if you are using prescribed sleeping tablets. May cause mild drowsiness which will affect your ability to drive or operate machinery. Do not take if you are pregnant or breastfeeding.

Peppermint *(Menthe piperitae)*

Peppermint contains an essential oil rich in menthol. It has antiseptic and painkilling properties and is also widely used to relieve flatulence, indigestion, nausea and other symptoms of I.B.S. Peppermint essential oil improves digestion by stimulating the secretion of digestive juices and bile, and also relaxes excessive spasms of the smooth muscle lining the digestive tract. While mild symptoms of I.B.S. are helped by drinking peppermint tea, more severe symptoms benefit from taking peppermint oil capsules that are enteric-coated to prevent the release of peppermint oil until it has reached the large bowel. These are available over the counter, or on prescription.

Dose

Enteric-coated capsules containing 0.2 ml: one or two, three times daily between meals. Treatment may produce a warm, tingling feeling in the back passage due to some of the essential oil not being absorbed. This is not harmful and will usually disappear if you cut back on the dosage you are taking.

Do not take peppermint during pregnancy, or if you are also taking homoeopathic medicines as it is believed to inactivate them.

Psyllium *(Plantago psyllium)*

Psyllium seed and husks are a highly effective, natural and gentle fibre source used to treat constipation in I.B.S. Their effectiveness derives from a mucilage present in the seed husks that swells to between eight and fourteen times its original volume when mixed with water. In the intestines, psyllium forms a laxative bulk that gently scrubs the bowel and absorbs toxins and excess fats.

DOSE

Take 1 to 2 tablespoons with water, twice a day.

Siberian ginseng *(Eleutherococcus senticosus)*

Over 1000 scientific studies show Siberian ginseng is effective in help-ing the body to adapt and cope during times of stress. Siberian gin-seng is used extensively to improve stamina and strength, particularly during or after illness. It seems to help the body adapt when under physical or emotional stress and boosts immunity. When given to 13,000 workers at a Russian car factory, the number of days off work due to health problems dropped by a third. Siberian ginseng – and related roots such as Korean ginseng *(Panax ginseng)* and American ginseng *(Ginseng quinquefolium)* – are useful herbal supplements to take when you are feeling under the weather, stressed or suffering from a relapse of symptoms.

DOSE

Take 1–2 grams per day. Occasionally, up to 6 grams daily is recom-mended. Choose a brand that is standardized to contain more than 1 per cent for eleutherosides. Start with a low dose in the morning at least 20 minutes before eating. If increasing the dose, work up slowly and take two or three times per day.

Siberian ginseng is best taken cyclically by those who are generally young, healthy and fit. Take daily for two to three months, then have a month without. Most people begin to notice a difference after around five days, but continue use for at least one month for the full restorative effect. Those who are older, weaker or unwell may take their doses continuously.

Take on an empty stomach unless you find it too relaxing, in which case take it with meals. A few people do find Siberian ginseng too strong, and it may affect their ability to sleep. If this happens, take the last dose of the day before your midday meal.

No serious side-effects have been reported, but do not use (except under medical supervision) if you are pregnant or breastfeeding, if you suffer from high blood pressure, a tendency to nose bleeds, heavy periods, insomnia, rapid heart beat (tachycardia), high fever or congestive heart failure.

Silicol gel

Silicon is one of the most common elements on Earth, coming second only to oxygen. It makes up 40 per cent of the Earth's crust and is found in a variety of substances including brick, cement, glass, quartz, emerald, silicon chips and even non-stick frying pans. The foods with the richest content include wholegrain wheat, potatoes and unprocessed barley, oats and rye.

Although silicon in its pure form is biologically inactive, it is now recognized as an essential trace element. In its soluble (colloidal) state, silicic acid, it is essential for normal growth and development.

Colloidal silicic acid can be helpful in treating the symptoms of I.B.S. It comes in the form of a gel which, when taken internally, reduces symptoms of bloating, flatulence and irregular bowel habit, especially diarrhoea. It has also proved helpful in the more serious bowel problems, ulcerative colitis and Crohn's disease.

As well as protecting the intestinal tract, silicic acid can soothe mouth ulcers and inflamed gums (gingivitis). It lines the stomach, absorbs toxins and irritants, and protects an inflamed stomach lining from self-digestion with stomach acid. It is therefore effective in the treatment of acid indigestion (gastritis) and heartburn due to acid refluxing up into the gullet (reflux oesophagitis). It is safe to use during pregnancy.

Intestinal problems helped by silicic acid include:

* I.B.S.
* Oral thrush
* Intestinal Candidiasis
* Nausea
* Diarrhoea
* Gastritis
* Reflux oesophagitis
* Flatulence

- Mouth ulcers
- Gingivitis

DOSE
Take 30 ml per day, diluted with fruit juice if preferred.

Valerian *(Valerian officinalis)*

Valerian is one of the most calming herbs available, and is used to calm nervous anxiety, reduce muscle tension, stimulate appetite and induce a refreshing night's sleep. Valerian contains a number of unique substances (such as valeric acid and valepotriates) that are thought to act together in synergy to produce significant, positive effects on stress. It is also used to relieve symptoms of I.B.S., intestinal colic, cramps, period pains, migraine and rheumatic pains.

DOSE
Take 250–800 mg, two to three times a day. Select standardized products containing at least 0.8 per cent valeric acid.

Valerian is not addictive and does not produce a drugged feeling or hangover effect, as it promotes a natural form of sleep.

Do not take if you are using prescribed sleeping tablets or if you are pregnant or breastfeeding. Valerian may cause mild drowsiness which will affect your ability to drive or operate machinery.

Medical herbs for specific problems

FOR PAINFUL BOWEL SPASM
Herbs with a natural anti-spasmodic effect include:

- Chamomile
- Lemon balm
- Peppermint
- Valerian

For constipation
Herbs with a natural laxative effect include:

* Aloe vera
* Dandelion root
* Ginger
* Flaxseed (bulking and lubricating)
* Psyllium husks (bulking laxative)
* Goldenseal

For diarrhoea
Herbs with a natural anti-diarrhoeal effect include:

* Slippery elm
* Goldenseal

Goldenseal helps to normalize muscular action in the bowel, and is therefore also advised by some practitioners to treat diarrhoea as well as constipation in I.B.S.

For bloating
Herbs that can ease gaseous distension and help bowel movement include:

* Angelica root
* Aniseed
* Cardamom
* Cayenne
* Chamomile
* Coriander
* Dandelion root
* Fennel
* Ginger
* Peppermint
* Thyme

Vitamins and minerals

Diet should always come first, but if you have I.B.S. and are unable to eat a balanced and widely varied diet, a complete vitamin and mineral supplement will act as an important nutritional safety net. Some researchers even believe that food sensitivity, which may trigger symptoms of I.B.S., is more likely if you are lacking certain vitamins and minerals.

Choose a supplement that contains as many vitamins and minerals as possible at around 100 per cent of the recommended daily amount (RDA). Although there is no guarantee that this will improve your I.B.S. symptoms, it will certainly guard against the common nutrient deficiencies and help to optimize your overall health. It may also prevent some of the common, niggling health problems linked with mild vitamin and mineral deficiency. Common symptoms linked with deficiency of vitamins and minerals include:

- Lowered immunity
- Poor wound healing
- Scaly skin
- Brittle nails and hair
- Premenstrual syndrome
- Constipation
- Inflamed gums
- Nerve conduction problems
- Muscle weakness
- Mouth ulcers
- Sore tongue
- Cracked lips
- Feeling tired all the time

To get the optimum level of nutrients from food, you need to:

* Eat food that is as fresh as possible, preferably home- or locally-grown
* Eat foods grown using organic farming methods where possible – these are usually significantly more expensive weight for weight, but not when measured by nutrients per pound
* Eat as much raw fruit and vegetables as possible
* Eat more whole grains, nuts and seeds
* Steam vegetables lightly or use only a small amount of
* water when boiling
* Reuse juices from cooking vegetables in sauces, soups or gravy
* Keep your use of processed, pre-packaged, convenience foods to a minimum

CHAPTER 18

Lifestyle changes and complementary therapies

You can make changes to your lifestyle that can help to improve symptoms of I.B.S. Following the guidelines below can make a significant difference:

1 If you smoke, do your utmost to stop, and try to avoid passive smoking. The gut contains receptors that are sensitive to nicotine and cause the bowel to constrict, making symptoms worse.

2 Get plenty of sleep. When you are rested, it is easier to stay relaxed and to cope with the stresses and strains of everyday life.

3 Take regular exercise, especially outdoors. As well as burning off stress hormones, exercise stimulates production of the body's own natural painkillers (endorphins and enkephalins). Exercise can reduce the discomfort of I.B.S., improve constipation, boost your overall mood and help you feel better in yourself. Exercise also hastens bowel emptying and can relieve bloating and distension. Aim to exercise for at least half an hour, three times per week.

4 Try to avoid unnecessary stress. The bowel also contains receptors that interact with stress hormones and make spasm and diarrhoea worse. We will look at stress in more detail below.

Stress and I.B.S.

Keeping a 'stress diary' will help you to monitor the causes of stress in your life so that you can attempt to do something about them. Try to fill in your diary immediately after each stressful event – don't leave it until later or you will forget exactly how you felt. Here is an example:

Date	Time	Situation	Feelings	Response	Future Remedy
Tuesday	9 a.m.	Overslept	Stressed	No breakfast	Set back-up snooze alarm
	9.30 a.m.	Late for work	Worried	Drove too fast	Leave in plenty of time
	10 a.m.	Stuck in traffic on way to meeting	Frustrated. I.B.S. pain started	Tried classical music	Leave in plenty of time
	6 p.m.	Super-market crowded	Hot and flustered	Rushed out forgetting to buy some things	Shop when store is quiter or order on line

At the end of a week, go back over your diary and try to identify your main sources of stress and how much control you have over them. Think about your habits and consider whether any are making things worse. For example, do you always shop on a Friday evening when the supermarket is unbearable? Do you always leave things to the last minute so you run out of time?

Look at your diary and try to pinpoint:

* Your main sources of stress
* How much control you have over these stressful situations
* Whether the stressful situations are likely to be long-term or short-term
* How stress makes you feel
* How stress affects your symptoms of I.B.S.
* How you are going to achieve more periods of rest and relaxation

---

BREATHING EXERCISES

We rarely think about breathing as it is an unconscious action. Stress will quickly change your breathing pattern, so that you over-breathe or hyperventilate with quick, irregular, shallow breaths. As a result, you will inhale too much oxygen and exhale too much carbon dioxide, causing an imbalance of gases in the lungs. This makes the blood too alkaline, leading to dizziness, faintness and 'pins and needles' in the face and limbs. This, in turn, creates panic and a cycle of anxiety. Fast, shallow breathing sends messages to the brain that you are under stress and keeps the body on 'red alert'. Habitual hyperventilators may also experience chest pains, palpitations, sleep disturbances and other physical symptoms, including those associated with I.B.S.

Research has suggested that chronic anxiety can be caused by hyperventilation rather than hyperventilation being a symptom of anxiety itself. Use the following exercises to control your breathing in situations where you feel stressed. They only take about two minutes to perform and nobody will notice you are doing them.

When feeling generally tense

* ❋ Sit back in your chair/car seat
* ❋ Drop and widen your shoulders by moving your arms
* ❋ Expand your chest and fill your lungs as far as possible
* ❋ Breathe in and out as deeply as you can, being aware of the rise and fall of your abdomen, not your chest. Repeat five times without holding your breath
* ❋ Continue to breathe regularly, getting your rhythm right by counting from one to three when breathing in and from one to four on breathing out

---

When panic rises
Use this exercise when you feel panic overwhelming you. It will help your tension subside and enable you to regain control.

- When the feeling of panic starts to rise, say 'STOP' quietly to yourself
- Breathe out deeply, then breathe in slowly
- Hold this breath for a count of three, then breathe out gently, letting the tension go
- Continue to breathe regularly, imagining a candle in front of your face. As you breathe, the flame should flicker but not go out
- Continue breathing gently, and consciously try to relax – let your tense muscles unwind and try to speak and move more slowly

GENERAL RELAXATION

Sit down quietly for an hour with a book or magazine. Use an aromatherapy diffuser to fill the air with the scent of a relaxing essential oil (such as chamomile or lavender). Have a candlelit bath to which a few drops of a relaxing aromatherapy oil has been added.

DEEP RELAXATION

For a deep relaxation exercise, which tenses and relaxes different muscle groups to relieve tension, set aside at least half an hour. This exercise is especially beneficial after a long soak in a warm bath.

1 Find somewhere quiet and warm to lie down. Remove your shoes and loosen tight clothing. Close your eyes and keep them closed throughout the session.
2 Lift your **forearms** into the air, bending them at the elbow. Clench your **fists** hard and concentrate on the tension in these muscles.
3 Breathe in deeply and slowly. As you breathe out, start to relax and let the tension in your arms drain away. Release your

clenched fists and lower your arms gently down beside you. Feel the tension flow out of them until your fingers start to tingle. Your arms may start to feel like they don't belong to you. Keep breathing gently and slowly.

4   Now tense your **shoulders and neck**, shrugging your shoulders up as high as you can. Feel the tension in your head, shoulders, neck and chest. Hold it for a moment. Then, slowly let the tension flow away, breathing gently and slowly.

5   Now lift your **head** up and push it forwards. Feel the tension in your neck. Tighten all your **facial muscles**. Clench your teeth, frown and screw up your eyes. Feel the tension on your face, the tightness in your skin and jaw, the wrinkles on your brow. Hold this tension for a few seconds then start to relax. Let go gradually, concentrating on each set of muscles as they relax. A feeling of warmth will spread across your head as the tension is released. Your head will feel heavy and very relaxed.

6   Continue in this way, working next on your **back** muscles (providing you don't have a back problem) by pulling your shoulders and head backwards and arching your back upwards. Hold this for a few moments before letting your weight sink comfortably down as you relax. Check that your arms, head and neck are still relaxed too.

7   Pull in your **abdomen** as tightly as you can. Then, as you breathe out, slowly release and feel the tension drain away. Now push out your stomach as if tensing against a blow. Hold this tension for a few moments, then slowly relax.

8   Make sure tension has not crept back into parts of your body you have already relaxed. Your upper body should feel heavy, calm and relaxed.

9   Now, concentrate on your **legs**. Pull your **toes** up towards you and feel the tightness down the front of your legs. Push your toes away from you and feel the tightness spread up your legs. Hold this for a few moments, then lift your legs into the air, either together or one at a time. Hold for a few moments and then lower your legs until they are at rest.

10 Relax your thighs, buttocks, calves and feet. Let them flop under their own weight and relax. Feel the tension flow down your legs

and out through your toes. Feel your legs become heavy and relaxed. Your toes may tingle.

11 Your whole body should now feel very heavy and relaxed. Breathe calmly and slowly and feel all that tension drain away.

12 Imagine you are lying in a warm, sunny meadow with a stream bubbling gently beside you. Relax for at least 20 minutes, occasionally checking your body for tension.

13 In your own time, bring the session to a close.

Complementary treatments for I.B.S.

An increasing number of doctors in the UK are starting to combine the best of complementary medicine within their work. A recent survey of over 1200 GP partnerships found that around 40 per cent provided NHS patients with access to some form of complementary therapy, of which acupuncture and homoeopathy were the most common. An estimated 25 per cent had made NHS referrals for complementary therapies.

The following complementary therapies have helped many people with I.B.S. Just as with orthodox medicine, however, all treatments will not suit every individual, so it is a question of trial and error to find one that suits you.

ACUPUNCTURE

Acupuncture is an ancient therapy based on the belief that life energy (chi or qi – pronounced 'chee') flows through your body along different channels called meridians. This flow of energy depends on the balance of two opposing forces – Yin and Yang – a balance easily disrupted through factors such as stress, emotions, poor diet and spiritual neglect. It is this disruption of the flow of energy through the body that is believed to produce symptoms such as intestinal spasms.

There are 12 main meridians. Half of these have a Yang polarity and are related to hollow organs (such as the gut). The other six are Yin and relate mainly to solid organs (such as the liver). Along each meridian a number of acupoints have been identified where chi energy is concentrated and can enter or leave the body. Traditionally,

365 classic acupoints were sited on the meridians but many more have now been discovered – around 2000 acupoints are illustrated on modern charts.

By inserting fine needles into specific acupuncture points, blockages are overcome and the flow of chi is corrected or altered to relieve symptoms. Fine, disposable needles are used which cause little, if any, discomfort. You may notice a slight pricking sensation, or feel an odd tingling buzz as the needle is inserted a few millimetres into the skin. The needles are usually left in place for up to 20 minutes, and may be twiddled periodically. Sometimes, a small cone of dried herbs is ignited and burned near the active acupoint to warm the skin. This is known as moxibustion.

The best-known effect of chi manipulation is in pain relief (local anaesthesia). Research suggests that acupuncture causes the release of natural, heroin-like chemicals that act as painkillers. Acupuncture can be effective in treating the symptoms of I.B.S., including constipation, diarrhoea and cramping pains.

Acupressure is similar to acupuncture, but instead of inserting needles at selected points, the meridians are stimulated using firm thumb pressure or fingertip massage. The best-known example of acupressure is shiatsu massage.

AROMATHERAPY MASSAGE

Abdominal massage is often beneficial in getting a constipated bowel moving, relieving wind and distension, or easing pain associated with diarrhoea. You can visit a qualified practitioner or carry out the massage yourself (see the following guidelines). You may find it helpful to apply alternating hot and cold compresses to your abdomen first to stimulate the local circulation. Some therapists also recommend that, 20 minutes before you start the massage, you drink a glass of hot water containing a few drops of ginger and fennel essential oils and sweetened with honey.

Selecting essential oils

To make an aromatherapy massage oil, you will need a carrier oil, such as almond or grapeseed. To 30 ml (1 tablespoon) of the carrier oil, add 10–20 drops of essential oil. The best oils to use for someone with general I.B.S. symptoms are rosemary and marjoram, separately or blended, to which a little oil of black pepper or fennel can be added. Other essential oils are also useful, depending on specific symptoms. These are listed below.

Note: Substitute rose oil for rosemary oil if you have high blood pressure, and avoid fennel oil if you suffer from epilepsy. Do not use aromatherapy oils if you are pregnant or if you suffer from any medical condition other than I.B.S., without first seeking advice about which oils are safe for you to use.

FOR CONSTIPATION:
* Black pepper (use sparingly)
* Cardamom
* Cedarwood (do not use during pregnancy)
* Fennel (do not use if you suffer from epilepsy)
* Ginger
* Lemon
* Patchouli
* Peppermint (do not use during pregnancy)
* Rosemary (do not use if you suffer from epilepsy)
* Sandalwood

FOR WIND AND DISTENSION:
* Cardamom
* Coriander
* Dill
* Peppermint (do not use during pregnancy)
* Spearmint

FOR DIARRHOEA:
* Basil
* Chamomile

- Lavender (do not use during first three months of pregnancy)
- Lemon
- Marjoram (do not use during pregnancy)
- Orange
- Peppermint (do not use during pregnancy)

FOR COLICKY, LOWER ABDOMINAL PAIN:

- Chamomile (do not use during first three months of pregnancy)
- Clove
- Cypress (do not use during pregnancy)
- Eucalyptus
- Ginger
- Lavender (do not use during first three months of pregnancy)
- Neroli
- Patchouli
- Peppermint (do not use during pregnancy)
- Rosemary (do not use if you suffer from epilepsy)
- Thyme (do not use during pregnancy)

Once you have blended your oils, you are ready to massage your abdomen:

1 Place the container of diluted oil in a bowl of warm water to heat it gently so it is comfortable to use on your skin.
2 At least an hour after last eating, lie down in a warm, quiet room with the curtains pulled. Expose your abdomen, but make sure you have a blanket or similar over your legs and chest to keep you warm.
3 Place some warmed oil on your hands and gently massage around your abdomen. Move in a clockwise direction, starting on the lower right-hand side by the groin, just above your pubic hair. Massage with slow, circular movements, pressing as deeply as you can without causing discomfort. Work your way up to the lower ribcage, across your upper abdomen and down the left-hand side to your groin again. All together, the massage should last around 15 minutes. It may be easier for a partner or relative to do this for you.

HOMOEOPATHY

Homoeopathy is based on the belief that natural substances can boost the body's own healing powers to relieve symptoms and signs of illness. Natural substances are selected which, if used full-strength, would produce symptoms in a healthy person similar to those they are designed to treat. This is the first principle of homoeopathy, that 'like cures like'.

The second major principle is that increasing the dilution of a solution has the opposite effect of increasing its potency i.e. 'less cures more'. By diluting noxious and even poisonous substances many millions of times, their healing properties are enhanced while their undesirable side-effects are lost.

On the centesimal scale, dilutions of 100^{-6} are described as potencies of 6c; dilutions of 100^{-30} are written as a potency of 30c, etc. To illustrate just how diluted these substances are, a dilution of 12c (100^{-12}) is comparable to a pinch of salt dissolved in the same amount of water as is found in the Atlantic Ocean!

Homoeopathy is thought to work in a dynamic way, boosting your body's own healing powers. The principles that 'like cures like' and 'less cures more' are difficult to accept, yet convincing trials have shown that homoeopathy is significantly better than placebos in treating many chronic (long-term) conditions, including hay fever, asthma and rheumatoid arthritis.

Homoeopathic remedies should ideally be taken on their own, without eating or drinking for at least 30 minutes before or after. Tablets should also be taken without handling – tip them into the lid of the container or onto a teaspoon to transfer them to your mouth. Then suck or chew them; don't swallow them whole.

Homoeopathic treatments are prescribed according to your symptoms rather than any particular disease, so two patients with the same label of 'irritable bowel syndrome' who have different symptoms will need different homoeopathic treatments.

In the UK, you are entitled to receive homoeopathic treatment on the NHS. If your doctor decides it is appropriate, he or she can refer you to an NHS doctor at one of five NHS homoeopathic hospitals, or at an NHS homoeopathic clinic. If your doctor refuses to refer you, he or she should be able to discuss the decision with you to explain why they do not feel it is appropriate. You can then request a second opinion. The British Homoeopathic Association publish a useful guide called 'How to get Homoeopathic Treatment on the NHS' *(see Useful Addresses)*.

Alternatively, you can consult a private homoeopathic practitioner or buy remedies direct from the pharmacist. Although it is best to see a trained homoeopath who can assess your constitutional type, personality, lifestyle, family background, likes and dislikes as well as your symptoms before deciding which treatment is right for you, you may find the following remedies helpful. If there is no obvious improvement after taking the remedies for the time stated, consult a practitioner. Don't be surprised if your symptoms initially get worse. Persevere through this common reaction to treatment – it is a good sign and shows the remedy is working.

For constipation with little desire to open the bowels:
Alumina 6c
(Take every two hours for up to 10 doses.)

For constipation with spasm and strong urges to open the bowels:
Nux vomica 6c
(Take every two hours for up to 10 doses.)

For constipation with large, hard, dry, crumbling motions:
Bryonia 6c
(Take four times a day for up to five days.)

For diarrhoea with flatulence or burning in the rectum and anus:
Aloe 6c
(Take hourly for up to 10 doses.)

For diarrhoea with anxiety and stress:
Argentum nit. 6c
(Take every half hour for up to 10 doses.)

For diarrhoea with anal itching or soreness plus foul-smelling wind:
Sulphur 6c
(Take every half hour for up to 10 doses.)

For alternating constipation and diarrhoea, with flatulence, colicky pain and passing mucus in the stools:
Argentum nit. 6c
(Take four times a day for up to 14 days.)

For colic with exhausting diarrhoea and excessive flatulence:
China 6c
(Take every 15 minutes for up to eight doses.)

For nausea, tearing pains and watery stools with mucus and loss of appetite:
Colchicum 6c
(Take four times a day for up to 14 days.)

For profuse diarrhoea with burning or colicky abdominal pains, restlessness, anxiety and chills:
Arsenicum album 6c
(Take every 15 minutes for up to eight doses.)

For green-tinged diarrhoea with abdominal rumbling and stomach cramps that are worse in the morning:
Podophyllum 6c
(Take every 15 minutes for up to eight doses.)

For profuse, strong-smelling, burning diarrhoea and an increased sensitivity to temperature changes:
Merc. sol. 6c
(Take every 15 minutes for up to eight doses.)

For simple diarrhoea associated with I.B.S., especially if symptoms are brought on by drinking coffee:
Psorinum 6c
(Take four times a day for up to 14 days.)

For griping bowel pains, which improve when doubled up:
Colocynthis 6c or 30c
(Take four times a day for up to 14 days.)

For sudden, colicky or shooting pains (especially on the right-hand side of the abdomen) that may be accompanied by bloating and are made better by doubling-up, or applying warmth and made worse by cold:
Mag. phos. 6c
(Take every five minutes for up to 10 doses.)

For bloating and distension, especially after eating or when constipated:
Lycopodium 6c
(Take every half hour for up to 10 doses.)

For back pain and a sense of spasm and coldness round the umbilical region with or without nausea or diarrhoea:
Terebinth 6c
(Take four times a day for up to 14 days.)

For I.B.S. symptoms, especially violent vomiting and diarrhoea, associated with cramps in the calves, headaches and menstrual problems or during pregnancy:
Verat. alb. 6c
(Take every four hours for up to seven days.)

After completing a course of homoeopathy, you will usually feel much better in yourself with a greatly improved sense of wellbeing that lets you cope with any remaining symptoms in a much more positive way.

BACH RESCUE REMEDY

Bach Rescue Remedy is a blend of flower essences prepared according to homoeopathic principles. It contains five flower essences preserved in brandy: cherry plum, clematis, impatiens, rock rose and star of Bethlehem. Rescue Remedy is useful for acute recurrences of symptoms that leave you feeling unable to cope, and to reduce the physical and emotional symptoms of stress and chronic illness, such as I.B.S. Add four drops of Rescue Remedy to a glass of water and sip slowly, every three to five minutes, holding the liquid in your mouth for a while. Alternatively, place four drops directly under your tongue.

HYPNOTHERAPY

Hypnotherapy can be effective in relieving the symptoms of I.B.S. Research shows that it can significantly reduce abdominal pain and distension, encourage a regular bowel and improve general wellbeing after just a short course of treatment.

In one study, a gastroenterologist and hypnotherapist together studied 32 patients with severe, refractory I.B.S. After eight weeks of half-hour hypnotherapy sessions, the sufferers achieved a stable improvement in symptoms. The hypnotherapist asked sufferers to place their hands on their abdomen and induce feelings of warmth and comfort in this area. He then made several suggestions related to symptom reduction and control over gut function. This was reinforced with visual imagery, and self-hypnosis tapes were provided for daily use. Overall, patients found that their abdominal pain and distension went from being moderate–severe to only mild or even non-existent.

REFLEXOLOGY

Reflexology is a relaxing complementary therapy based on the principle that points in the feet – known as reflexes – are indirectly related to other distant parts of the body. Massage over these reflexes can detect areas of tenderness and subtle textural changes that help to pinpoint problems in various organs, including the gut. By working on these tender spots with tiny pressure movements, nerves are thought to be stimulated that pass messages to distant organs and relieve symptoms. Some people with I.B.S. have found reflexology helpful as it can relieve fatigue and a number of stress-related symptoms such as tension, migraine, breathing disorders, premenstrual syndrome and digestive problems.

At the end of each session you will usually feel warm, contented and relaxed. You can buy a variety of mats, rollers, shoes and brushes that stimulate the reflexes for self-help, but if you are unable to visit a therapist, you and a friend can easily learn to give each other a relaxing foot massage. Use a little aromatherapy oil to make the experience more therapeutic.

1 Hold your partner's foot in both hands for a few moments, then start stroking the top and bottom of the foot by moving both hands from the toes towards the ankles and back again. Use a light, firm motion and repeat several times to warm the skin.
2 Holding the foot firmly, gently rotate and rock it from side to side and round and round throughout the whole range of movement at the ankle.
3 Holding the foot still, use your thumbs to apply gentle but firm pressure over the sole of the foot. Cover the whole sole with small circular movements of your thumbs.
4 Repeat the circular thumb massage on the top of the foot and the base of the toes.
5 Holding the foot under the heel with one hand, use the other to gently grasp all the toes and flex the end of the foot up and down.
6 Gently squeeze and massage each toe one at a time, starting with the big toe.
7 Finish by stroking the foot a few times as before. Let your fingers slide towards the ends of the toes. Hold the toes for a few moments then gently place the foot on the ground and cover with a towel while you repeat the massage on the other foot.

VISUALIZATION

Visualization harnesses the power of the imagination. It boosts self-confidence, promotes relaxation and can ease stress-related symptoms. It relies on the power of suggestion and positive thought to visualize a desired outcome and is similar to meditation, but less structured and easier to perform. It involves entering a relaxed state and allowing your own inner thoughts (or someone else's voice) to guide you on a self-improvement quest or to take you to a quiet place of inner peace. When you feel an attack of pain coming on, try visualization to aid relaxation and relieve your distress. Stop what you are doing and sit down somewhere private and quiet, if possible. Guided visualization most commonly involves the use of a relaxation tape in which you are instructed on how to relax before imagining yourself somewhere pleasant such as:

* Walking through a sunlit forest glade, with the sound of gently running water and birdsong surrounding you while a cool breeze ruffles your hair.
* Swimming in a warm tropical ocean next to a white-sanded, deserted beach.
* Sitting in the sun on the veranda of a log chalet high up on a snow-crested mountain – breathe in the cool air and hear the soft drip of snow melting from the surrounding fir trees.

Unguided visualization uses the same elements except the journey is replaced by your own wandering thoughts. Imagine looking through a window, for example, and describe what you can see. Then allow your imagination to take you closer so you can see, hear, feel, touch and smell what is happening there. Explore the shapes, sizes, colours and positions of different objects to heighten your senses. Stay in this state for about 10 minutes and then bring yourself slowly back to everyday feelings.

A mandala can be used to assist your visualization or meditation. This is an intricate diagram used to represent the universe in Hindu and Buddhist traditions. A mandala usually consists of a series of concentric circles surrounded by an outer enclosure. These in turn may surround other geometric shapes containing the symbols or images of gods. Eastern mandalas are basically of two types, representing different aspects of the universe: the *garbha-dhatu* in which the movement of the eye across the mandala is from the one to the many; and the *vajra-dhatu* in which the eye moves from the many into one. Concentrating on the images on a mandala can help you achieve a guided visualization or a meditative state.

Symptomatic visualization

If a particular stress-related symptom such as bowel spasm and pain is troublesome, picture an image in your mind that represents that symptom and imagine it away. For example, visualize the bowel as surrounded by an iron band which gets progressively looser until it falls away.

YOGA

Yoga is a gentle movement therapy that uses posture, breathing techniques and relaxation to increase suppleness and vitality, calm the body, improve sleep and relieve stress-related symptoms. Like all therapies, it is best to receive training from a qualified teacher who will help you achieve mental control and the right yoga positions for you. Before starting:

* Check with your doctor if you have a back problem or high blood pressure
* Do not do yoga within an hour of eating – wait three hours after a heavy meal
* Empty your bladder and bowel
* Don't mix yoga with smoking, drugs or alcohol
* Wear comfortable, light clothing, which stretches easily

Breathing plays an important part in yoga as the breath is thought to embody your life force or *prana*. The following exercise is an example from the range of yoga positions that can help you achieve relaxation through posture and breathing.

The Triangle (Trikonasana) – alleviates anxiety and stress

1 Stand comfortably with your legs slightly more than shoulder-width apart, with your feet facing forward.

2 Breathe in, and raise your right arm alongside your right ear, stretching as high as possible. As part of the same movement, your right arm will follow over to the left, forming a graceful curve from your fingertips down to your right foot.

3 Breathe regularly and hold the position for 30–60 seconds.

4 Make sure you keep looking forward, not down, that your knees and upper elbow are straight, and that your body and feet are not twisted.

5 Return to your original position as you inhale.

6 Repeat the exercise again, this time moving to the right.

CHAPTER 19

Other bowel problems and diet

Symptoms of I.B.S., such as constipation, can lead to other bowel problems that can also be helped by making dietary changes.

Haemorrhoids

Haemorrhoids (piles) are dilated varicose veins that form in the rectum and around the anus when valves in the veins that usually prevent back-flow of blood give way under pressure. This is especially likely during straining if you frequently develop constipation through I.B.S.

Piles form soft, fleshy lumps that may remain inside the back passage or be visible outside. Swollen veins close to the anal opening are called external haemorrhoids, while those occurring higher up in the anal canal are known as internal haemorrhoids. They are also classified according to their severity:

* First-degree piles are confined to the anal canal and bleed only
* Second-degree piles prolapse (i.e. come out of the rectum) on opening the bowel but reduce spontaneously or can be pushed back in, gently, afterwards
* Third-degree piles persistently prolapse outside the anal canal

Symptoms of piles include a constant dragging sensation and bright-red bleeding which is sometimes copious (although rectal bleeding should always be reported to your doctor in case it is due to another, more serious cause). Haemorrhoids may also itch – especially if they are prolapsed and produce a mucus discharge. External piles sometimes become hard, intensely painful and dark purple-black in colour if the blood trapped inside them starts to clot (thrombosed pile). This usually resolves spontaneously over two to three weeks, but consulting a doctor who will anaesthetize the area and gently evacuate the clot through a small incision brings instant relief. If you suffer from haemorrhoids:

* Eat a mild, non-spicy, high-fibre diet and drink plenty of fluids.
* Use glycerol suppositories to ease motions and reduce straining; straining can also be reduced by leaning forwards from the hips when opening the bowels.
* Bath or shower every day using unperfumed soap and finish by spraying the area with cold water.
* Keep the area scrupulously clean to help stop itching – wash with unscented soap after each bowel motion and pat dry with a soft tissue. If necessary, keep dry using a hairdryer set on gentle heat.
* Wear loose cotton underwear, changed at least once a day.
* Avoid talcum powder.
* If you scratch at night, try wearing cotton underwear and even cotton gloves.
* Aromatherapy: try adding one drop of peppermint oil and two drops of chamomile to warm water (in a bidet or large, shallow, plastic bowl) and sit in the solution for five to ten minutes.
* Cypress, lemon and chamomile Roman essential oils are another helpful combination. If the area feels sore and burning, you can also add two tablespoons of bicarbonate of soda.
* Over-the-counter preparations (creams and suppositories) are available to relieve pain, itching and to numb the area. Ask your pharmacist for advice on which would suit your symptoms best.
* Herbal medicine: astringent ointments containing comfrey, horse chestnut or witch hazel are used; horse chestnut also strengthens supporting tissues around the veins. The seed and husks of psyllium are a safe and effective remedy for constipation and haemorrhoids (see page 201).
* Homoeopathy (take four times daily for up to five days):
    * For piles with burning, soreness and bursting feelings: Hamamelis

- With sharp shooting pains up the back: Aesculus
- With feelings of a full rectum: Nux vomica
- With itching and burning: Paeonia
- For feelings of heat, burning and itching when overheated, bleeding or associated with painless diarrhoea in the morning: Sulphur
- Acupuncture can be highly effective.
- Haemorrhoids can be shrunk by injecting them, tying them off with rubber bands (so they eventually drop off) or removed surgically.

Diverticular disease

Diverticular disease, or diverticulosis, affects most people in the Western world. The term simply means that small pouches have formed in the large intestine (colon) where the lining has herniated through the muscular outer layer of the bowel. This is thought to be caused by increased pressure such as straining, most commonly from constipation. Faeces may become trapped in the diverticular pouches and cause inflammation (diverticulitis) that needs treatment with antibiotics. If abdominal pain worsens, always seek medical advice.

A fibre-rich diet helps to stimulate bowel function, reduce constipation and decrease the chance of any pouches becoming infected and inflamed, causing diverticulitis. Eat as wide a range of fibre-rich foods as possible from wholegrain sources, fruit and vegetables, but increase your intake slowly so you don't develop wind and bloating from an initial fibre overload. To get maximum benefit, you should regularly vary the types of fibre in your diet. If taking fibre supplements, such as bran, ispaghula, psyllium or sterculia, vary them every month or so. Drink plenty of fluids, which are needed to help fibre swell and work effectively. Probiotic supplements containing bowel-friendly bacteria help to maintain optimum bowel function, while aloe vera juice and colloidal silicol gel (available from health-food stores) have a useful cleansing and soothing action on the intestines.

Anal fissure

An anal fissure is a tear at the anal margin. This can form when large, hard, constipated motions pass through, especially if the bowel action is rapid and violent. An anal fissure is intensely painful and causes spasms that make symptoms of I.B.S. and constipation worse. Your doctor may recommend a local anaesthetic cream to numb the area, drinking plenty of fluids and eating a high-fibre diet. If healing does not occur within a few days, a chronic fissure sometimes needs a simple treatment under general anaesthetic – the surgeon simply inserts several fingers into the anus and stretches the anal margin to overcome spasm. This is known as a Lord's stretch and works by temporarily paralysing the anal muscles so that the rested parts can heal. A special spray that encourages reheating anal muscles can also be prescribed if your doctor feels this will help.

Rectal prolapse

In extreme cases, constipation and straining may push a small portion of the rectal lining (mucosa) out through the anus, where it resembles a large, moist strawberry. This can usually be gently coaxed back into the rectum by a doctor using a lubricant and local anaesthetic. A high-fibre diet and drinking plenty of fluids will help to avoid constipation and encourage the prolapse to heal. If recurrent, the prolapse will need to be surgically removed or stitched back in place.

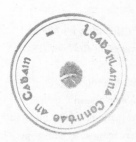

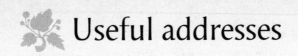

Useful addresses

Please send a stamped, self-addressed envelope if writing to an organization for information.

The British Allergy Foundation
Helpline: 020 8303 8583
www.allergyfoundation.com
For information about food intolerance.

British Dietetic Association
5th Floor
Charles House
148/9 Great Charles Street
Birmingham B3 3HT
Tel: 0121 200 8080
www.bda.uk.com
For information on state-registered dieticians.

British Digestive Foundation
3 St Andrew's Place
London NW1 4LB
Tel: 020 7487 5332

The British Society for Allergy, Environmental and Nutritional Medicine
Tel: 0906 3020010
www.bsaenm.org.uk
For information on food intolerance. Members are doctors with a specific interest in this field.

Coeliac Society
PO Box 220
High Wycombe
Bucks HP11 2HY

IBS Bulletin
Latest updates on diagnosis and treatment of I.B.S. produced for sufferers by a team of medical researchers. For details of subscription send an sae to I.B.S. Subscription Dept, Central Middlesex Hospital NHS Trust, PO Box 18, East Sussex TN6 1ZY.

Central Middlesex Hospital NHS Trust I.B.S. Research Team
Telephone Helpline: 0336 411286
Calls are charged at 39p a minute cheap rate, and 49p a minute at all other times.

Nutritionists
A list of nutritionists can be seen at www.nutsoc.org.uk

The Inside Story Monthly subscription magazine for anyone with food sensitivity or on a restricted diet. Recipes, product information, research and news reports, specialist articles, children's club and useful resources. Edited by Michelle Berriedale-Johnson
5 Lawn Road
London NW3 2XS
Tel: 020 7722 2866
E-mail: info@inside-story. com
www.inside-story.com

Wheatwatchers.com Antoinette Savill's website provides advice and information about wheat- and gluten-free products and diets. Savill's range of products is available by mail-order or from Waitrose supermarkets in the UK.

Women's Nutritional Advisory Service
PO Box 268
Lewes
Sussex BN7 2QN
Tel: 01273 487366
Advice and nutritional information for treating I.B.S.

Complementary therapies

British Acupuncture Association and Register
34 Alderney Street
London SW1V 4EU
Tel: 020 7834 1012
Information leaflets, booklets, register of qualified practitioners.

British Association of Nutritional Therapists (BANT)
27 Old Gloucester Street
London WC1N 3XX
You can obtain a list of registered nutritional therapists by sending £2 plus a large (A4) sae to BANT at the above address.

British Herbal Medicine Association
Sun House
Church Street
Stroud GL5 1JL
Tel: 01453 751389
Information leaflets, booklets, compendium, telephone advice.

British Homeopathic Association
27A Devonshire Street
London W1N 1RJ
Tel: 020 7566 7800
E-mail: info@
trusthomeopathhomoeopathy.org
www.
trusthomeopathhomoeopathy.org
Leaflets, referral to medically-
qualified homeopathic doctors.

**British Society of Medical and
Dental Hypnotherapists**
17 Keppel View Road
Kimberworth
Rotherham
South Yorks. S61 2AR
Tel: 01709 554558

Colonic Irrigations Association
50A Morrish Road
London SW2 4EG
Tel: 020 8671 7136

**Council for Complementary and
Alternative Medicine**
Suite 1
19A Cavendish Square
London W1M 9AD
Tel: 020 7724 9103
Details on a variety of techniques
and practices. Leaflets, booklets,
newsletter.

**General Council and Register of
Naturopaths**
Frazer House
6 Netherall Gardens
London NW3 5RR
Tel: 020 7435 8728

Institute for Optimum Nutrition
Blades Court
Deodar Road
London SW15 2NU
Tel: 020 8877 9993
I am impressed by this organization,
whose members obtain the DipION
qualification. A register of members
(many of whom are also BANT
registered) is available at
www.ion.ac.uk or you can find a
therapist in your area by contacting
ION at the above address.

**International Stress Management
Association**
The Priory Hospital
Priory Lane
London SW15 5JJ
Tel: 020 8876 8261
Information on stress management
and control. Leaflets, booklets,
counselling.

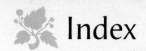

Index